Motivation for Current an

Endure Smarter Not Harder

"Consolidated wisdom from athletes who have been there and done that"

By: Grant Shymske

Edited and Foreword by: James Vreeland

Ryan:

Great work at nav!

I hope you get a lot out of this book.

Grant Shymske

Motivation for Current and Aspiring Endurance Challenge Athletes
Vol. 1 2

© Copyright 2013 by Grant Alexander Shymske

All rights reserved.

© Copyright Cover photography by: KO Amanzi

Photography

Dedication

I would like to dedicate this book first and foremost to my best friend, my battle buddy in life, my wife Chanelle, who makes everyday a great day worth living to the fullest.

I would also like to dedicate this work to all the GRT's out there who have become my friends, my family, and who have inspired me so much over the years. We have done amazing things together and there is still so much to do!

Motivation for Current and Aspiring Endurance Challenge Athletes
Vol. 1

Acknowledgements

Every one of the fantastic and inspiring athletes who both contributed to and influenced the writing of this work are owed my deepest thanks, without you this work would be worth so much less.

Robert Alban, Caitlin Alexander, Ben Anderson, Hailie Beam, Paige Bowie, Andy Cappelli, Lauren Cisneros, Harrison Lee Coale, Olof Dallner, Stephen DeToma, Ann Eckler, Troy Gayer, Dominique Gordon, Spencer Guinn, Chris Holt, Jeff House, Brian Johnson, David Kim, Eric Kling, KO Amanzi Photography, Todd Kruse, Candace Appleton Kuntz, Lou Lepsch, Tracy McGuigan, Christopher Meredith, Christian Nelson, Matt Ogle, Michael Petrizzo, Erin Hamilton Prindle, Tim Rosenberg, Richard Sanders, Martin Schmidt, Jason Spare, Greg Stroud, John Templeman, David Thomas, Adam Trevillian, James Vreeland, Mark Webb, Chris Way, and Dana Lynn Whitmore

Special Thanks

The entire GRT community, and the inspiring and motivating athletes amongst them pushing back the boundaries of the fitness and endurance world.

"Hard times make hard people." -Lou Lepsch

"Men wanted for hazardous journey. Low wages, bitter cold, long hours of complete darkness. Safe return doubtful. Honour and recognition in event of success." -Ernest Shackleton

---

"He who learns must suffer, and even in our

sleep pain that cannot forget falls drop by drop upon the heart. And in our own despair, against our will, comes wisdom to us." -Aeschylus

---

"Know Thyself."

- Inscription within the Temple of Apollo at Delphi

Foreword

The sport of endurance challenge racing is incredibly new, and as such, there simply hasn't been enough time for "the way" to success to evolve. How do you adequately train for races that could include anything from land navigation and ultra distance movements to memory games and extreme weather survival? To excel in these events you must train as hard as possible, plan heavily for the obstacles that you know will be in your path, and listen to the advice of those who have gone before you and conquered the challenges you wish to face.

Grant is an incredible resource for this all-important knowledge. He has either personally completed, or trained racers for most current competitions. Even more importantly than cleanly sailing through events, he has occasionally stumbled during the hardest races on earth. This has driven him to intensely study his physical training, mental preparation, and gear selection. His focus on both internal and external obstacles to victory has allowed him to conquer these previous blockers, complete the worst of the worst challenges, and earn his current placement as one of the top athletes in the field.

I have had the pleasure to compete with Grant on numerous occasions, and during one event the phrase "Hard times, make hard people." was used to describe the ordeal. This simple comment resonated with me, and explained in one simple sentence the different between those who attempt, and those who conquer this special breed of sport. Grant has been through the hardest events,

and heeding his advice will give you the strongest chance of

success in your own undertakings.

-James Vreeland - endurance athlete

Introduction

The world of adventure racing and obstacle course races has exploded in the past few years. This rapid expansion has resulted in a number of heavy hitting companies emerging as the standard bearers for difficulty and innovation in this newly minted 'sport'. While all of them are different in their own way, they center around the objective of getting people outside of a usual or expected setting, pushing some personal boundaries, and in the end allow participants the opportunity to surprise themselves with their ability to overcome their predispositions.

If you are like me then you do not want to simply participate in a chosen event, you want to dominate it! You may strike your friends as a little eccentric and a tad over competitive when it comes to activities involving a definitive 'winner'. This work is meant to be fuel for your fire and the world of endurance challenges will graciously accept your eccentricities and pay you back with an ever upward spiraling staircase of difficult events for you to test your farthest limits against.

One of the facets of these challenges that makes them so

hard and interesting is the variability not only between event brands but within the events themselves. These challenges can combine running, load carrying, rope climbing, swimming, dynamic lifts, neck deep mud, sleep deprivation, and hunger all in the same event! This multifaceted nature also makes these sorts of events somewhat overwhelming to prepare for, especially for the uninitiated. But because of this variability, any but the very best and most detailed 'how to' book (more like encyclopedia) could hope to prepare people completely.

So what to do? Well I don't have all the solutions (and that is sort of the point of this book) but I figure I can take a stab at helping out those interested by utilizing a learning technique that has never failed me yet: asking those who have gone before you for advice. You can study a task until your eyes itch but sometimes the best information comes from the person in front of you who just successfully completed the task without breaking a sweat.

What I wanted to do here is compile some wisdom from athletes who have been there, done that, and earned the t-shirt. I wanted to put it into a book because the place I usually got this kind of valuable insight was at or after the event in question, and of course by then it is far too late to implement any of those useful nuggets. So don't wait until you are sucking through it the hard way or worse yet sitting on the sidelines totally defeated; take the sagely advice from these experienced veterans and implement their techniques to create your success story.

Whenever possible I have interviewed and directly quoted the athletes themselves. However there are situations in life where you learn a valuable lesson worth passing on and yet failed to have an audio recording device at the ready. Because of this I have paraphrased and summed up lessons I have learned either by personal experience or acquired from others via some other circumstance than a recorded interview. Because I have felt they are worth passing on you can consider them my personal opinion on the subject at hand and affix whatever credit to the advice that you see fit.

Why endurance challenge? Well if this term seems delightfully vague, that's because it is. As I mentioned before these events are so varied in their structure that to be more specific would lead to an incredibly detailed and frankly over complicated book. And since I have already mentioned that the buck does not stop here, I want you to get what you can from this book quickly and move on to other learning/training experiences. So in order to simplify referring to events ranging from 5k mud runs, to quintuple IRONMAN's I will be from here on out generally referring to all of these events as 'endurance challenges'.

Storytelling is a method for communicating information and lessons that is as old as civilization itself. I love stories in a learning context and remember frequently searching for the oft provided 'analogy' in the lecture during my study in philosophy that would 'click' all the given information into place. I feel that learning through the telling of another person's story is a comforting and relaxing way to digest what would otherwise need to be ground through by repeated readings or droning lecture. Such is another reason why I wanted to include the quoted stories of other's experiences in this work whenever possible.

A Note on Method:

From the outset I wanted this work to revolve around inspiration. To that end it is not intended as a scientific work, nor is it intended to stake new claims in the worlds of exercise science or physiology. All the statements in this work are either taken from the direct experiences of those athletes quoted or of myself. Any additional claims or statements of fact are cultivated from non-fictional works by respected authors in their scientific fields and any information used has been tested by myself or one of the athletes here at least once. This is not an attempt at a claim to authority and encouraging skeptical exploration and inquiry is one of the primary goals of this work.

Rather, the athletes quoted in these pages are socially accepted within the small, and tight knit circles of extreme endurance athletes and their advice is rarely taken lightly. By gathering their wisdom in the setting of interesting and often humorous stories, I hope to give the seasoned competitor a great read and perhaps a take on things they had not considered before; and more importantly for the up and comer I hope to provide an interesting introduction to this fast paced and wild community and help them integrate in a way that makes their experience enjoyable to the point that they value the time spent and yearn for more.

Contents

Training

Full Spectrum Training

Hardening Your Body and Mind

Weathering the Storm of Doubt

Selecting and Testing Your Equipment

Active Recovery and Intelligent Event Approach

Nutrition

KISS

Be Skeptical

Eating for, and During the Big Event

Don't Sweat the Small Stuff

Friends and Battle Buddies

Why Are You Doing This Anyway?

Unconventional Families

Accountability

Some Extra Stories

Winter Death Race 2014

Making the Challenge more of a 'challenge'

Silly Man

Motivation for Current and Aspiring Endurance Challenge Athletes Vol. 1

The First Goruck Heavy

Bragg Heavy 2.0 AAR

Baptism By Fire

Back to Back to Back to Back Endurance Challenges

Final Thoughts

Source List and Recommended Reading

Training

Training is your key to success, in encapsulates everything you do (mentally and physically) to prepare for your event. Endurance challenges are not simple affairs and so showing up with a handful of practice runs and a trusty pair of running shoes is rarely going to cut it. All the events involve multiple disciplines of physical fitness, will be subjecting you to a number of psychological hardships and frequently have packing lists. These variables are part of what makes endurance challenges so interesting, especially to seasoned one-disciplined athletes; but it is also what makes them so chaotic to prepare for.

Full Spectrum Training

"Treat your body like you hate it and it will reward you." - Dan Plants

Extreme endurance challenges (as the name implies) are extreme and taxing on the body and mind. What this often means is that simply working on physical fitness alone will not be sufficient to allow you to perform at the levels that you would like. The term 'full spectrum training' is simply a succinct way of describing an approach to training where every aspect of your humanity is considered ranging from mental toughness to nutrition and skincare. This route of training can also be an excellent way to examine your daily habits and work to improve your overall quality of life as well as elite athletic performance.

"Train how you fight" is an Army mantra that has a lot of wisdom behind it and can be applied to so many endeavors in life. Simply put it means that you should train under conditions as similar to the event that you are training for as possible. While in some circumstances this can be impossible, putting in the effort can make a huge difference in your level of preparedness come the day of the event. Putting in the effort to practice the refit and repair drills you plan to implement during your event may be time consuming. However, it only takes one monumental error during an important event to make you realize that every aspect of your event left unpracticed is a chink in your armor begging fate to exploit it.

At the most physical level exercise science has found that 'like' exercises contribute only some of the same benefits as the one (or many) that make up the event. This means that substitute exercises and activities can be useful to help prevent overuse injuries and switch things up but in the end nothing truly replaces the real thing. While the constantly changing nature of these events prevents the kind of laser focused training that makes becoming an Olympic athlete so hard and rare, the principle of 'muscle memory' still plays a role. Practicing exercises or tasks that you know will be part of the event (even if you don't have the whole picture) can still give you an edge.

Is it likely that you are going to try and bring your mMP3 player to wear during your event? If the answer is no (and it should be for almost any serious endurance challenge that involves mud, the ground, or water) then it is a very good idea to train without using it. The mp3 player is a blessing to the workout community and provides stimulation and possible educational benefits for long drives and workouts alike. However, when dealing with psychologically challenging events where quitting is a source of DNF's it is not a good idea to tackle the event 'unplugged' for the first time in a while. Intense and uplifting music stimulates and occupies the mind during intense and draining workouts and can help you get numbers that you might not otherwise be motivated to achieve.

Going cold turkey on the tunes can be a shock to the system when you discover that the little demons in your head telling you to quit are much louder without death metal drowning them out. Learning how to 'live inside your own head' and like it there is an essential mental skill when dealing with events that actually try to make participants quit. You have to be attuned to your sense of purpose and precursors to emotional spikes and moods that can tip the balance between motivated determination and whimpering defeatism. Training without music will not solve all of these issues but going sans music will allow you to focus on your emotional states while training and better understand your particular states of mind and adjustable attitude.

Motivation for Current and Aspiring Endurance Challenge Athletes

Again and again one common factor that comes up when differentiating between those who finish an event and those that do not is time spent training. Time is one of those factors that people like to ignore because it is so unavoidable, it is one of the leading excuses given by those quitting work out regimens (namely not having enough of it), and is commonly cited as the reason for not training enough for extreme endurance events. The hard truth is that for the worlds most extreme endurance challenges the successful athletes will more often than not be the ones who trained the longest and most often.

If you are an American reading this then there are an uncountable number of factors vying for your time at any given moment. Careers, family, hobbies, cell phones, social media, and friends are only the tip of the iceberg. But the sad reality is that you can't buy or create more time in a day, you only have so much. What this means is that if one of your goals in life is to say win the Spartan Death Race or pass GORUCK Selection you are going to have to make sacrifices to the vices of everyday living.

One of the first pieces of advice I give to Selection/Death Race/Ultramarathon hopefuls is "Train like a man possessed", this usually elicits a half humorous smile but I mean it in the most literal sense. If you are focused on conquering one of the few top tier endurance challenges then that goal needs to occupy a constant and nagging place in your brain and its presence there should not inspire fear in you but rather a burning, passionate drive to prepare for success. People in your life should be regularly telling you to "Shut up" because you try to fit some aspect of your preoccupation into every conversation.

This goes double for the seasoned veterans. There are already OCR (Obstacle Course Racing) athletes out there who are on a year long 'circuit', a schedule planned out months in advance with events they want to attempt. If you are like this and one of those events on the list is a wholly different beast altogether then you are setting yourself up for failure. I have met and talked to many fantastically talented and insanely fit endurance athletes who drop out of top tier events because they are either still recovering from a previous event or they quit as to not injure themselves for a future event on the calendar. Such events need to be your sole focus, everything else can and will get in your way physically and mentally.

Friends and family will only suffer your all consuming passion for so long. there is a reason why intensely passionate and mission driven careers like the various branch's combat arms have such high divorce rates. Luckily if you are not foolish your endeavor should not last so long for that type of damage to your personal life to come about. If you maturely plan your goal out you should dive down the rabbit hole just long enough to prepare for and conquer your dream and then (win, lose, or draw) take a break to focus on personal matters before jumping back on that horse for either another shot or the next big challenge.

Frequently people don't even realize that time is a factor. It tends to be a variable that sits in people's blind spot. Bewildered VW's (Voluntary Withdrawals) will shake their heads in dismay and repeat that they trained during all of their spare time and can't for the life of them think of what else they could have done. The truth in fact is that these people have far more 'spare time' than they think; if you cut out social media, TV, and going out to eat the hours just start piling up, and all of them should be used for training.

I tell individuals beginning to train for top tier events to use the mantra "What am I doing to prepare for my event right now?" and if the answer is nothing then do something about it. All of this is applicable for events on the same level of difficulty, it is just amazing how much time you have if you limit yourself to communicating with your immediate family and face to face contact.

So how do you find the time? There is no perfect answer to this question but the short story is that it takes effort; you really have to make this integration something you enjoy and you cannot be afraid to be a little different from those around you as a consequence. One tactic I have had significant success with is hobby integration. As a chronic student and occasional writer I am necessarily reading all the time; the one major drawback of reading however is that it usually calls for sitting on your butt. Luckily as a side effect of long car rides with my dad growing up I knew about and enjoyed audio books.

The audiobook industry has come a long way in the last few years and as a result you can find a truly impressive selection of fiction and nonfiction titles to suit your purposes. Listening to my books while at the gym combined two very enjoyable activities for me and thus made this time both very productive for me as well as something I very much looked forward to everyday. Learning to pay attention to the book while keeping track of reps can be a little disorienting at first but if you stick with it you will soon find that it becomes second nature.

Another method for maximizing your time is simply a more extreme version of the habits trainers try to integrate into the lives of those desperately trying to get back into shape. Sometimes athletes start to believe that 'real exercise' only happens at the gym or on a run/bike/swim. The reality is that there are lots of great training opportunities sandwiched in between busy times in your day that you simply have to creatively exploit. Walk/jog from your car to where you are going, plank when you read or knock out twenty five push ups every time you turn the page.

Instead of just throwing the ball for your dog to fetch why not chase the dog around the yard a couple of times? If you have an athletic dog you would be surprised how much of an agility/sprint workout this can be. Your only limit here is your own imagination. If exploited properly you'll find just how much training time is available to you throughout your average day. Plus you get to enjoy that shocked expression you elicit when asking for walking directions to a location more than fifty feet away.

Training style and approach are intensely individual choices for an athlete to make. With both successful and floundering athletes loudly recommending every exercise program under the sun , is there really one right choice for the aspiring endurance athlete? The short answer is no; training for success comes in many and varied forms but has underlying values and commonalities that go beyond the 'brand name' of the workout style. As with so many other things in life knowledge is power, and knowing your objective, yourself, and your resources makes the difference between a successful lifestyle switch and a temporary fad your buddies will make fun of you for later.

Some of the more popular endurance challenges have become synonymous with certain fitness styles. Spartan Race and GORUCK are often associated with CrossFit (though unofficially), while IRONMAN and marathons have had many similar training plans published specifically for those working towards competing in them as well those looking to improve their results in future races. In many cases the underlying exercise science and expert opinion of seasoned veterans would indicate these associated workout styles to be the best course of action for a potential athlete looking into the specific race concerned; however, there is certainly some wiggle room that successful athletes can and do explore.

A lot of what is advisable for an athlete focusing on a specific endurance challenge is based on their goals. If you are new to trying triathlons and are only concerned about finishing then you have a variety of inexpensive and high quality training plans and exercise disciplines to choose from. However if you are experienced in the field and are looking to win your next race then spending the extra money on a personal trainer who specializes in that event could be well worth your money.

Extreme endurance athlete Christian Nelson has done more Tough Mudder's than most (far, far more) with impressive results to his name. When looking to branch out to other events like GORUCK he decided to stick to his guns and maintain more or less the same training plan with slight modification added in, he explains:

"I do very traditional workouts. Cardio like Elliptical machines, running, and stationary bikes, coupled with weightlifting. Before my first Tough Mudder I used the "Tough Mudder" workout they had posted on their site, which was comprised of pull ups, kettlebell stuff, mountain climbers, etc. At least once a week I try to get a few miles under a weighted rucksack, hiking up local 'mountains'. I would really like to get into CrossFit, but my life schedule doesn't permit it."

As an already experienced endurance athlete, Christian was able to assess his new interest and decide that it required many of the same strength and endurance conditioning proficiencies that he already trained for and so only tweaked his training to accommodate the added GORUCK variable of rucksacks with bricks. This is an important lesson for those who are already athletic and wish to take on endurance challenges; many of the underlying physiological requirements are similar and all that may be required is a sober assessment of the expected intensity level and special circumstances and an effort to adjust training to address these variables effectively.

For the individual who is relatively new to the athletic world and is not well entrenched in a personal training routine, the recommended workout programs might just be what you need to kick start your experience. Training consciously and continuously takes practice and benefits from initial structure that is hard to make up on your own. So for the beginner it is much easier to follow the recommended workout routines until you have built a fitness relationship with yourself and the style that you most enjoy. Once you get the handle of things you can then make modifications and enhancements in order to both improve your performance and prevent yourself from dying from boredom.

Christian Nelson mentions the stability and opportunity for enhancing changes when talking about his implementation of Tough Mudder's proffered workout routine:

"The workout on their site at the time was diverse and a great place to start. It hit a lot of body groups. I eventually found that it wasn't hard enough so I would add weight where I could and did the workout twice. Other than that I'd say it would work well. Since then I've been more concentrated on lifting and gaining muscle. For no other reason than seeing big numbers on the weights I guess. And to look good in Ranger Panties."

The fact is that if you are just getting into the endurance challenge community (or even the athletic lifestyle in general) you should not expect miracle performances right off the bat. In fact the only thing you should be worrying about at first is making it through your chosen event in one piece. This means that any pre-conceived notions of effective fitness regimens or workout styles garnered from the internet or health magazine should be stowed in the back of the mind until you have objectively experimented with recommended approaches and thoroughly evaluated whether or not they are effective for you.

Female endurance athlete Dana Lynn Whitmore was turned

on to CrossFit through peer recommendations and decided to see

what it was all about. A CrossFit gym is as much a community as it

is a place to work out. Participants receive coaching and feedback

from instructors as well as motivation and encouragement from their

peers. It also aims to be a resource for 'full spectrum fitness' in that

a participant who puts in the time and effort will see gains in all

areas of fitness and even diet if they choose to follow the gym's

recommendations. Dana explains the motivation she received and

the focus that it gave her to make significant lifestyle changes:

> "It wasn't until CrossFit and GORUCK that I started
> becoming serious and methodical with my workouts.
> Goals to lean up, not just look good, but to become
> stronger. I started planning meals that were
> balanced. I started eating to fuel my body rather than
> just to fill my belly."

The type of physical conditioning required to shine in the

most extreme endurance challenges is not something that is

attained overnight, it is not a weekend retreat so to speak, it is an

'all the time' thing. As was mentioned before, making fitness your

hobby is one of the only ways you can look at training for these sorts of events without seriously disrupting your usual freetime activities. This means that you need to learn how to enjoy the time you spend at the gym (or wherever you train).

If you cannot get over looking at training time as an inconvenient necessity that you must pay lip service to in order to get through your chosen event then this lifestyle is almost certainly not for you. Get your finisher's award, start some interesting conversations looking at it with friends, and be content that that is as far as you will go in that world of dedicated athletes. This may seem harsh, but the reality will sink in post event. You will either hang up your t-shirt and cross the event off your bucket list, or you will almost immediately start looking for another event in your area and adjusting off of lessons learned from your first endeavor.

There are a number of approaches to making training time something you look forward to. One is to use it as a more or less peaceful time of reflection in your day. It is a widely known fact that regular exercise reduces stress and enhances mood, by coupling this with a positive outlook and I mindset that your gym time is 'me time' where you can burn away your stress and 'reset' can make that time very pleasant and beneficial to your everyday life.

When I use this approach in my training I also double my

benefits by listening to audiobooks on my MP3 player. This could be just for relaxation if you like listening to books and working out at the same time (some people don't, you'll have to give it a shot and find out for yourself). I personally write in my non-gym free time so I find great satisfaction in 'killing two birds with one stone' by researching through my headphones while working out at the same time. Workout buddies might think my sporadic scribblings on random napkins and sticky notes are my way of tracking my reps when in reality I am marking time for direct quotations I utilize later in my work.

Another approach is to look at your training time in a similar light to the way dedicated sports fans approach watching the game. Get competitive with yourself and your gym buddies, use your time training to compete with yourself and others in a positive way in order to achieve greater gains and faster times. This approach can be an even greater stress reliever, especially if you tend to be a competitive person as you can vent those tendencies at training where it is very beneficial instead of in less appropriate areas of your life.

A technique that can (and should) be applied to both of the aforementioned approaches to fitness is variety. Switching up your workout by incorporating a cornucopia of different exercises not only prepares you more effectively for the kinds of things that will be demanded from you during endurance challenges but will also speed your strength and endurance gains far faster than exclusively training a few disciplines ever could. Tony Horton is fond of saying "Variety is the spice of fitness." and it is absolutely true that changing things up benefits both your mind and body alike.

All around grizzled and generally tough as nails athlete Jason Spare makes variety a point in his training, he talks about how it preps him for the wide variety of events he tackles each year:

> "I try to keep in shape year round, all the time. I balance strength and endurance training to stay ready for anything. I never do the same workouts, with the exception of the main 4 strength movements: deep squat, deadlift, standing press and bench press. Around those, I utilize Crossfit, kettlebells, TRX, body weight training and conditioning drills. Throughout, I believe in running, as well. Harden the body for anything. The closer to an event, I'll tailor my workouts to suite the event: more heavy rucking, weight vests, unpleasant environmental training

(water and elements) etc…"

Like I quoted before: variety is the spice of fitness. Not only can you capitalize on muscle confusion, you will also keep yourself interested in working out. Well planned and timed cross training can greatly improve performance in even the most specific performance activities. Also, the more diverse you are willing to be the more likely you are to relate to friends and family and the activities they do will then become time together.

If you are an aspiring endurance athlete and are just beginning to explore the world of training then I highly suggest getting as much information and researching things as much as possible. If you are serious about setting your goals high initially I would also suggest hiring a sports specific personal trainer to help you develop safe, well rounded, and focused workouts and training habits. Whatever you do, try not to get sucked into the large proportion of aspiring athletes who want to go fast and save a buck by following some downloaded workout program with no knowledge of form, recovery, or safe workout techniques. People who do this disproportionately end up sitting out their season due to injury.

If you are an elite athlete training for an unconventional endurance challenge it can sometimes be hard to find help with your unique goal. For this reason it is imperative that you have a solid knowledge base in exercise science and your own limitations because you may find yourself as your own personal trainer. This also means that you are likely a hard charging, type A, meat eating, extrovert who drives too fast. Controlling your own ambitions to within a tolerance that keeps crippling training injuries at bay is going to be the name of your game because you are blade running down into a lifestyle that no licensed trainer is going to want to risk their reputation on.

Marine Corps Gunnery Sergeant and well qualified endurance challenge athlete Robert Alban chose to "Go full retard" when training up for GORUCK Selection class 013 in Washington DC. Trainers would not touch him and probably thought he was nuts, though he likely flirted with injury many times he took the risk and of the 21 candidates who showed up for that class, he was the only one to be selected... In his words:

"Training for GRS was a blast – nothing was ever too crazy or outlandish. When I told a potential coach I wanted to do a ½ IronMan Triathlon followed the MCM (Marine Corps Marathon), which was 2.5 weeks before my GRS (GORUCK Selection), she promptly stopped her assistance with training plans. So I created my own plan: I continued my triathlon training and sprinkled in weighted rucks, 'special' GRCs (GORUCK Challenges) with double bricks, no food, no sleep, a 100-pound sandbag 'team weight' (which my friends all thank me for…haha), two GRCs 'back to back', and/or staying awake for 48+ hours.

High intensity training w/ extra weight constituted a lot of my training. Two-a-days were the normal part of my workout regimen; my caloric and protein intake skyrocketed. I did a lot of these training events together with friends, and they made for fond memories. Needless to say, I started Selection in subjectively the best shape of my life."

Again, even with the amount of experience and background knowledge Robert was bringing into his training he was still taking some substantial risks. However sometimes in life you may deem that the goal you are trying for is worth the risk; Robert did, and he achieved his aims as a result.

Diversifying your training and workouts will also help you prevent overuse injuries that can chronically plague athletes who specialize too much. Endurance athlete Hay Lee always has variety in mind even when time does not allow for heavy volume in training, occasionally changing things up will keep things interesting and avoids injury.

> "I'm always partaking in different events, so I attempt to fit a variety of training in. I get bored with doing the same challenges back to back, just like I get bored with the same workouts. In a perfect world, I would be able to fit CrossFit, swimming, yoga, running, biking and martial arts into one week. Typically, I only have the time/make the time for Crossfit and running."

A word of caution when the endurance challenge lifestyle gains traction in your life. While training can be tapered with some focus and reasoned reflection in your physical conditioning habits, signing up for too many events has a way of gaining a life of its own and takes significant willpower to beat back. This is what happens when the advice to 'capitalize on your free time' goes a bit too far.

Signing up for more than you can handle can have a number of negative effects on your life. For one it will interfere with your professional and family life, causing unnecessary stress and strain that no one needs. For another thing it will contribute greatly to your chances of 'burning out' where athletes far over do it and end up forgetting why they got into this hobby to begin with. In short, endurance challenges are meant to give you a sense of achievement and the opportunity to have fun pushing your boundaries; overdosing on this eliminates the fun and blunts any thoughts or feelings of achievement.

When volunteering at some of the more extreme endurance challenge events I often come into contact with DNF's who have over scheduled their lives. These people will be some of the fittest and hardcore individuals you will ever meet and yet they drop out of the harder events because they have bitten off more than they can chew in the long run. Sometimes their drop will be because of a severe flare up from an injury sustained during last month's event that they have simply not taken the time to get healed properly or bothered to go see a specialist about. Other times the story will be the pile up of minor aches and pains that begin to chip away at their resolve because they have another race the following month that they don't want to have to drop out of because of x, y, and z.

This is a great example of too much of a good thing. I have personally met athletes who really enjoy the culture and don't mind doing similar events regularly because of groups of friends they meet there habitually. This works for them because they cycle on and off between doing the events and volunteering to support; on top of that the events are similar or the same so they have the opportunity to more or less adapt to them physically.

The problem children are the endorphin junkies who sign up for the hardest and most grueling events they can find and space them out barely 30 days apart. These events by their definition are impossible to fully 'adapt to' or can be with nothing less than total focus in training for the better part of the year. Trying to tackle this sort of schedule leads to overuse injuries and severe burnout. The best advice I can give is try to have fun whenever possible, take breaks, and when you want to tackle a top tier event then make it your sole and undivided focus until it is done and over with.

There is a fine line between hardass and dumbass, and I talk about it here because it relates to training and what you bring to your event. There is a habit I see too often at events where participants make things extra (unnecessarily) hard for themselves intentionally. Whether it is putting twelve paving stones in your ruck instead of the required six bricks (massive weight difference) or going on a long trail run without water breaks, this 'going hard to be hard' mentality is often misplaced in my opinion.

My philosophy has always been to train your ass off and then crush your event according to its rules. If the event is easy, all the better! That means that my training was successful and I need to start looking for a harder event. I don't try to do the same event again after having my friend

fire an arrow into my hip so it can be 'hard'. You are being

an ass doing this in one of two ways. If the event is

individual then you are skewing your time/standing and not

doing as well as possible by the rules of the event. And if

the event is team oriented then so much the worse because

not only are you asking to screw yourself but you absolutely

are screwing your team by not presenting with 100% output

available.

Some events are not easy under any circumstances,

for anyone. Whether it is because the event is just so

massive that it pushes the conceivable boundaries of

human capabilities, or the event has no fixed distance (for

instance the maximum number of laps run in 24hrs). In such

cases your training and nutrition need to be spot on and in

addition to this you must seek special knowledge or

assistance in refining your technique as 'gutting it out' in

such monumental undertakings is simply not possible. Peak

endurance athlete Olof Dallner describes his approach to

training for his quintuple IRONMAN. With a twelve mile

swim, a 560 mile bike ride, and a 131 mile run, such an

event redefines what is physically possible, let alone difficult:

"I did push myself outside my comfort zone for training. Biking 560 miles is one thing. You can coast on a bike. Swimming and running is different. I knew I had the running distance down. Swimming was different though. Swimming 12 miles takes training and commitment. You can just push through but then you will also completely deplete yourself and there is a long way to go after the swim. So I trained quite a lot of open water swimming.

My approach to training for this is having focus weeks. One week I'd focus on swimming, the next biking, and the running. Distance wise I think you should be able to do the distance your training for in a week. That is, if you're training for a marathon you should be able to total 30 miles in a week. If you're training for a 100 miler you should have 100 mile weeks.

I didn't quite live up to this on the bike part due to lack of time. Then I occasionally do longer overnight runs and and bike trips and back to back events. For example I'd bike overnight Friday, sleep very little, sleep very little next night too, and then race a half ironman Sunday morning. It's important to see how you react during nights. Your body wants to shut down and sleep and you need figure out how to trick your brain to continue."

Such distances and times are far outside the human ability to adapt to completely through training meaning that no one will sail through such a thing at least until we get really good at genetic engineering. Until then you will not only have to endure a massive amount of discomfort in the face of sleep deprivation and hunger but also you will have to perfect the skills to do each event well so as to give your endurance a chance at lasting to the end.

One aspect of modern unconventional endurance challenges is the sheer variety of exercises, functional tasks, and just plain odd things you might have to do during them. Traditional training models for endurance events involve volume, volume, and more volume with a little speed/power and skill drills sprinkled in for a little variety. Old school marathon and IRONMAN athletes will simply pound away at their events for countless hours a week. In preparing for a modern endurance challenge this type of approach will do a few things, it will make you very good at one or two aspects of a 15-30 aspect event, it will make your body rigid and unadaptable, and it will generally grind your joints and ligaments to powder.

There is a lot of emerging data and exercise methodology that centers around functional fitness and diversifying your workouts to incorporate power, speed, agility, balance, and accuracy to train a well rounded athlete. One aspect of the old paradigm remains though with a little tweaking and that is specific training in the movements you will be performing during your event, however with a focus on technique and form rather than massive volume and repetition. Endurance challenge athlete David Thomas describes his workout approach to specific aspects of GORUCK Selection, the event he happened to be training up for at the time:

"Most of my training consisted of body-weight training and specific activities I knew we would be doing – bear crawls, burpees, crab-walks, etc. There are some training guides available. I didn't use any one specifically. I took ideas from different sources. I had a pretty good base because I do a lot of HIIT (High Intensity Interval Training) normally. I am always conscious of core stabilization and strengthening. I did incorporate some strength training — squats, deadlifts, and shoulder presses.

These seemed to cover the bases as far as where I might need strength. I would also carry 40 lb dumbbells around the house and hold them overhead a lot. I would wear my ruck or a 40 lb weight vest around the house as well, just to get used to bearing weight. If I was just standing around or brushing my teeth I would hold one leg straight out for as long as I could — building strength, stability, and learning to manage pain. I did yoga, which I think made a huge difference. I tried to do it 2 or 3 times a week. Not only was the stretching beneficial, but learning to control my breathing and relax was extremely valuable in handling the cold water."

As we have already discussed, there is no better training for an upcoming event than a 'dress rehearsal'. Getting out into conditions and terrain similar to those in which your chosen event will occur in will give you all kinds of insight into how you can adjust your training and equipment to become better prepared. Endurance athlete and as of this writing sole female finisher of GORUCK Selection Paige Bowie shares some insight on her use of 'dress rehearsals' in her preparations for GRS:

"I followed the plan, but I also added some beach PT sessions. I only did it a couple times, just to get comfortable with it. One night it even rained, which was perfect. Some of my advice for this thing is to actually do the stuff you know you're going to get. It sounds easy but it can be hard to just go do it. Go do it, and in all the proper gear. A lot of things are different in the sand: how your gloves work, how push-ups feel, bear crawls, etc. A friend came out to the beach and put us through the ringer for what seemed like 5 hours. What seemed like five was in fact only two. That was a reality check. But the experience helped when it came time to doing it in Selection. Beach PT still really, really sucks, but I knew I was going to attack the water.

One last thing that worked for me: take as many variables out of the equation as you can. Of course you want to be ready for anything, but be smart and minimize the uncertainty. Tweak your gear until you have it dialed. If you live where your event is, think about what they might do. You know you'll be in the water. Look around you and think, what is the hardest, craziest thing they could have me do? Then go do it because the cadre are evil and creative! I even looked up the moonrise times, and the weather. All the little details make a difference."

A common saying that is often misused by the lazy as an excuse to not prepare is "Everyone has a plan until they get punched in the face." My retort to this when it is used incorrectly is "Unless you plan to get punched in the face." and that is exactly what Paige and every other successful top tier endurance athlete that I have spoken to lives by. To expect chaos and rehearse contingency after contingency will put you in a position to immediately react and push on while others are reeling.

People like to think they can 'stay loose' and go with the flow but the fact of the matter is when you are physically exhausted and mentally fatigued your brain is going to be operating only on basic functions and the only thing that will save you in these instances are procedures you have drilled into yourself so much that they have become second nature. This is where your 'what if' drills pay for themselves in quick reaction times and insights that end up saving your butt when things go wrong.

Hardening Your Body and Mind

Toughness can describe many aspects of an athlete both physical and mental. One of the endearing qualities of toughness is that it has to be acquired through experience; there is no 'magic pill' that can give it to you. A lot of what can be described as 'tough' is really experience that allows the person in question to confront a situation with little or no fear. This experience gives clarity, focus, and the ability to drive towards the foreseen objective instead of becoming caught up and pulled under on the way to it.

As I mentioned there is no easy way to acquire physical or mental toughness, you simply need to put yourself in similar situations or train to the level of intensity that the event or situation you are preparing for dictates. By mentally rehearsing your actions and physically replicating them you can get your brain used to the experience which will go a long way towards preventing you from over focusing (tunnel vision) on small and inconvenient details of the experience. The goal here is to allow (through exposure) your brain to distinguish and 'edit out' insignificant details in the task at hand and devote total focus to what is important.

As GORUCK's Cadre Bert said, "One constant fear for

candidates is cold water... once we put them in they always start dropping like flies". There is some kind of primal fear in entering freezing cold water that can turn the toughest athletes into whining children. It doesn't get better with time and the initial shock can even be fatal for people with certain heart issues. I have personally participated in more than one event where a deciding factor in making it to the end centered around the participant's ability to stick it out in freezing water. When preparing for World's Toughest Mudder Christian Nelson remembers not fearing the grueling miles ahead, but the weather and the water:

> "With WTM I pretty much knew what to expect. It was going to basically be a Tough Mudder course over and over, so I wasn't too nervous mentally. I was more afraid of the weather. I knew it would be cold, and I knew there would be water. So my preparation was mostly with gear and just accepting the fact that it was going to be a cold night. I noticed the night before while out with friends I was more quiet than usual. More in my own head than usual; I was getting focused on what was ahead."

For events that are long and restrictive (under time constraints that prevent rest, drying off, or regular first aid) there are often preparations that serious and successful athletes make in order to better prepare their bodies to endure the challenge. Often these preparations are not part of any kind of exercise routine as the environment of the gym or track does not necessitate their use and so many training athletes are left to seek advice or do their own research (or learn the hard way through experience on the course). Unconventional prep like spraying your feet with extra strong antiperspirant or daily walks on asphalt in bare feet to toughen them while not proven, have worked enough for some seasoned athletes for them to swear by the practice.

Short of learning through trial and error after having your feet obliterated in your inaugural thirty-plus mile adventure race, the smart athlete will try to learn from other's experience. However, as with any medical or physical adaptation that is developed in highly subjective circumstances ("It worked for me! I swear") one should always look for proven studies or other such research that provides substance for your peer's personal claims. If nothing else just try techniques out in training, do not wait until your event to try something off the wall with no prior testing. Doing so is only asking to ruin your day.

There is usually one common denominator when it comes to preparing for the abuse that your mind and body will go through, and that is that you will not be near home. You might be able to shed your filthy clothes and hop in a steamy shower if you abuse yourself at home but most people will have to travel to their event of choice, many going great distances. In general the rich kids have it made, it is a pretty safe rule that your comfort level and the luxury of your recovery are inversely correlated to the amount of money you hope to save on your trip. So if you are a hardcore athlete on a budget then just make peace with baby wipe baths and back seat sleeping bag arrangements. The good news is that if you put out and did well in your event you likely will not care all that much, and if you are good at making friends you might even be able to crash in someone's hotel room.

One of the biggest 'hardening factors' that separates the men from the boys so to speak is the experience of knowing your body and how it communicates with you. It is a fact that people get injured at endurance challenges. It is also a fact that nowhere near as many people get injured as you might think. Also, the ratio of people who drop out for perceived injury or its immediate onset vastly outnumber the people who are actually hurt. Because of this, being an athlete who can tell if they are really hurt or just 'hurting' is a huge advantage worth cultivating.

Seasoned SOF veteran and co founder of The Professionals Group Lou Lepsch has two endearing quotes he teaches by. "There is no magic pill." and "Hard times make hard people." Both of these sentiments are applicable to the endurance challenge world. Some people might be gifted with a naturally high mental resilience but experience counts for a lot here. So while I will never discourage people from 'reading up' and 'doing their homework' this is one area where you just need to put in the time pushing your limits. By getting outside your comfort zone and training the areas you are bad at you will build your tolerance for discomfort and adversity. There is no easy way around this, you need to put in the time and 'pay your dues' so to speak.

I am not a doctor, all I can give are observations and those should not be taken as de facto evidence that your personal experience will exactly match what I have seen. That said I will cautiously put forward that injuries taking people right out of an event are trauma oriented (falling or being fallen on, serious allergic reaction, bear attack etc.). Most athletes that were responsible and entered the event healthy and properly rested/recovered from other events and training do not generally develop non traumatic, event ending injuries (overuse injuries mostly) during the course of that event. Overuse injuries generally come from people who trained like demons up until hours before the race or those who overschedule endurance challenges to the point that they overload their bodies.

Take solace in the fact that you rarely if ever run into anyone permanently hobbled by an event. Most of your struggling participants have previous injuries (car accidents are the most common ones I run into) or congenital illnesses. If the gene pool didn't decide to kick you in the shin from the get go then remind yourself that the most dangerous (life, limb, or eyesight) part of your whole event is the car ride getting there. This is one reason why many of the top finishers in the hardest endurance challenges are older individuals. Amongst other things they simply are not freaked out by life the same way a nineteen year old is, stress and hardship does not get to them nearly as much.

One of the most important pieces of equipment (if not the most) that you will have with you at any event will be your feet. Nothing puts a stop to an endurance run or race time faster than a severely blistered foot. Even for people with the pain tolerance and perseverance to push through such a predicament it is still not the optimal circumstance and it is certainly one that an athlete can take steps to prevent. However, foot care and toughening techniques are not part of your average personal training curriculum and there are certainly no pieces of equipment at the gym designed to toughen your tootsies.

So what is an interested and eager athlete to do? There are a couple of things that you should do in order to find out what foot preparation methods work best for you. The first is to do your research! You have made the choice to pursue endurance challenges that take physical exertion and personal endeavor well beyond the realm of normal activity so the path of least resistance is already closed to you. This means learn everything you can about the event you are interested in, watch videos, read write ups, and talk to as many veterans as possible. Be honest about your abilities and take seriously advice from people who match the same physical and mental characteristics as you. There is nothing more pathetic that an athlete who gets hit by a major issue on the course that they arrogantly laughed off before the event.

Another option is to take a test run in an event that is less intense than the one you want to tackle. There are plenty of 5k distance 'fun mud runs' out there and they tend be both plenty cheap and usually for good charitable causes. Use these kinds of events to test out new gear, some new prep plan, or friends and relative who you want to convince to join your cause. If a 5k mud run is your goal then just get out there and run a pre-measured 5k distance and throw some potential wrenches in like jumping in a pond and running through some rough 'off road' terrain in order to replicate some of the aspects of the actual course.

The last mandatory preparation for your event is to talk to and otherwise seek advice from as many veterans of the event as possible. I am assuming here that your objective is to make it through the event at all costs and that you are trying to do your personal best performance wise. If however, you want the unexpected and don't care about performance then you can disregard this advice but still be sure to read and abide by the safety points listed on the respective event page. Advice is variable and subjective so it is important to get second and third opinions when possible. Also, be sure that the person you are getting advice from has actually participated in (and finished) the event in question.

Another bonus piece of advice is to not rest on your laurels if you happen to have a record of successful events in your past. It is easy to forget in hindsight all the extra time and effort you put in to be successful on that first attempt. Just because you have finished a particular event in the past does not mean that the unexpected can't happen to you or that the operators of the event will keep things conveniently similar to your previous experiences. Dana Lynn Whitmore emphasizes this point in discussing her foot care preparations:

> "I thought I had the feet thing taken care of until my last GORUCK Heavy. I never have problems with my feet during challenges, and I got through two other Heavy's with no blisters or hot spots. Philly completely changed that. So, really this answer encompasses two important things. One, never get so comfortable with your ability to perform that you

start forgetting things you need to prepare.

For example, I always spray my feet with Arrid XX Dry, put my toe socks on and finish with a light wool regular sock. Before Philly I put my toe socks on and realized I forgot to spray my feet and I really didn't feel like taking them off to spray my feet. I paid BIG TIME for that. My feet were thrashed. Two, train your mind to be prepared for anything. Nothing is out of the question during these events. I learn something different about myself at each one. Whether it is something I need to work on during training, or about team work."

She participated in the same type of event three different times in three different places and although GORUCK prides themselves on stressing the unconventionality of their events, Dana's mind still managed some complacency. It can happen to anyone and especially to those who have gotten just beyond the realm of 'beginner's luck'. The key here is to experiment and test to find out what works for you and then stick to it. No matter how many events you have under your belt you are still human and your body will only need more maintenance as time goes on.

Toughening up for the rigors of an extreme endurance challenge is an imprecise and highly variable endeavor. As with equipment selection the process can be very individualistic and encapsulating the hardships of sleep deprivation, hunger, and extreme heat or cold into pre event training can be very difficult. This is another instance where experience is one of the best teachers you can recruit to your cause. It is also why athletes that are successful in in the hardest events have usually participated in similar events of lesser severity. Just like with dialing in your fitness, you will come to find that certain areas come naturally to you while others present intense challenge. Learning to identify these weak points in your mental game and developing mechanisms to help you cope is a key step in overcoming the extreme adversity imposed on athletes in the most extreme events.

Matt Ogle describes some of the things he has learned in training his mind and body to endure extreme adversity. You can identify in his outlook where the line exists between the already experienced and the unknown:

"I haven't previously done much of anything in

terms of physical toughening, but after getting a few blisters (foot) during a normal challenge this past weekend, I'm going to spend some time working on toughening up my feet including barefoot walking and using Tuf Feet, which one of the Selection finishers, I believe it was Tim Erwin, said he used with success.

Nagging problems are a big issue. You try as hard as you can to be 100% when you start an event like Selection, but with the intensity and volume of training necessary to be prepared for an event like that, it's got to be very difficult to be truly 100%, and you never know which injury will be okay and which will turn into a catastrophic problem, so I'm guessing its a bit like a roll of the dice.

I'm not really sure if you can train for things like hunger and cramping and other issues that would arise during an event like that and at the level they will hit during such an endeavour without having previously done an event similar to it. It's hard to replicate those issues in training without destroying the body, like you would during Selection. I went without food during my challenge this past weekend to see how I dealt with a lack of food in that situation, but of course that's nothing like the duration and intensity of Selection.

To develop that thought a bit, my sense is that trying to train for every eventuality in Selection is a fool's errand. I think you have to realize that you can never be totally ready, be okay with that, and be ready to get hit with a lot that you haven't necessarily directly prepared for. I know I need a plan, and I also know that cadre, especially Bert, likes to find and attack people's plans ("Everybody's got a plan until they get smacked in the mouth"), so I'm trying to keep my plan as simple as possible to allow for flexibility and adaptability during the event.

I've got a fairly flexible plan that's still developing, but seems to make decent sense at the moment: 1. Get my body as ready as I can. 2. I'm a very competitive person, so turn the event into Me vs

Cadre, and that basically one of us will win the event. I'll win by finishing and they'll win by making me quit and there are no ties. and 3. Attack each task with enthusiasm and vigor. That's all I've got so far, and like I said, it's developing, but I doubt it will change too much. I guess the only other thing I've got in mind is to be as grey as possible. Keep my head down and my mouth shut and let other people get the attention as much as is possible."

Many times the best thing you can do when preparing to face unknown adversity is to get your mind set on it as best you can. Then focus on solving problems as they arise as opposed to dreaming up hypothetical ones as you go. Focusing on the 'what if's' during the event will simply distract you and drain your willpower. Regardless of how well prepared you are mentally for the unknown it is still a dangerous place; performance feeds on routine, practice, and confidence.

The unknown is the proverbial 'wrench thrown in the works' by definition you will not be ready for it. The lack of experience often leads to novel feelings in both body and mind, and many of these feelings are mistaken for immanent injury or otherwise life threatening conditions. This case of mistaken danger or 'freaking out' is the cause of innumerable dropouts and DNF's in extreme endurance challenges. A cool head and a flagrant disregard for pain and misery are one's only hope in such unknown circumstances.

While the debate rages on regarding the spectrum of appropriate applications for minimalist footwear, their benefit in training is quite solid. While my personal opinion is that when the day of the event arrives it is game time and any gear that is meant to challenge you or 'build' strength translates into "Makes it harder to win".

This is antithetical to my entire mindset of utterly destroying the event and the competition. Anything short of the unhonorable or blatant cheating is permitted as far as I'm concerned and that means footwear that lets me work easier and go farther while burning less calories is where I am going to look. That said I am all about toughening my body and building bone and tendon strength in training.

While I always looked at it as a bit of a gimmick that I am paying more for 'less' of a shoe, many athletes have experienced great benefits from minimalist footwear. I personally skipped the shoes and just trained barefoot, you necessarily can't do as much this way but you would be surprised how fast your feet toughen up when you walk a few miles of sidewalk in bare feet day after day. Also try to hop on the treadmill in bare feet from time to time, run slower than you normally would and put yourself on a slight grade and you're in for a good cardio and foot toughening combo. Ultra endurance athlete and minimalist footwear advocate Jason Spare discusses why he likes it:

> "As far as feet, my feet are strong due to lots of running, barefoot running and flip flops! Yup! I'm a huge opponent of over corrective shoes. Build up the bones, connective tissue and callouses for running and endurance events. Environment: I try to keep myself exposed to the environment that I'll be participating in. I try to expose myself to what I hate, or perceive as a weakness."

Little techniques and tricks of the trade can come in really handy when you are dealing with extreme fatigue or sleep deprivation. Everyone is affected differently and to different intensities with regards to sleep deprivation probably involving underlying genetic circumstances. But building your cardiovascular endurance as well as your experience with the fatigued condition can help you to 'function' better in such a state.

For the most part though training to the point of extreme fatigue will not necessarily allow you to be more alert but rather you will make peace with how your body reacts to that condition and it will freak you out less. Along with this you will develop some tricks to keep yourself as sharp as possible when you need it and how to rest and recharge when you do not.

Extreme ultra endurance athlete Olof Dallner shares the techniques he used to focus and rest during his quintuple IRONMAN spanning monumental distances over a great length of time:

> "I engage my brain in specific tasks. During this race I keep track of the other athletes and try to race against them. That is not because I'm trying to be very competitive, I do it so that my brain stays focused and engaged. If you're not racing you could focus on something else. I sometimes find a certain point, like a top of a hill and I put all of my focus on reaching that hill and I don't think about anything else. During this race I ended up sleepwalking during

one of my last laps and I was literally falling over, losing a lot of pace. So when I got to my crew I just sat in a chair and slept for 3-5 min and then just stood up and continued. It's amazing how you can reboot your brain with such a short micro nap."

During endurance challenges lasting twelve hours or longer (and almost certainly in events over twenty four hours) participants can experience the warped world of intense sleep deprivation. This is of course assuming the event in question does not permit rest breaks or requires you to take none in order to be competitive. Something that can't really be 'trained' (in the context of getting better at staving it off) sleep deprivation or 'droning' as it is sometimes called can often be a hinderance to a competitive athlete, an asset to others, and a trippy wild time for everyone involved.

Generally divided into two categories (acute and chronic) the type of sleep deprivation you will experience during endurance challenges falls squarely into the 'acute' category unless your event is a week long or something. This means that your lack of sleep will be a singular event as opposed to accumulating over a lengthy period of time. This is a good and bad thing. Good because you will be less likely to experience the long term issues and heightened disease susceptibility faced by chronically sleep deprived people.

Bad because you will be aware of how much you are being affected and will experience more intense symptoms in a shorter time period. The good news is that as a rule endurance challenges don't have you operate heavy machinery or juggle newborns or anything potentially devastating. You'll generally just have to learn to prevent yourself from freaking out and fight for at least enough awareness to prevent yourself from wandering off a cliff.

Seasoned endurance challenge athlete David Thomas has experienced his fair share of 'zombie time', here he recounts an experience he had during GORUCK Selection:

"We were given instructions about the trail and water-points and headed out. First water-point seemed to take a couple hours to get to, with the second about the same. Then it was a REALLY long time before seeing any sign of a water-point or even civilization for that matter. I began to think this was the wrong trail. Now my mind was clearly playing tricks on me.

I saw 09 walk through a tunnel on the trail. He stopped at the end and I could see him speaking to someone sitting on a rock. I thought "Great, that's a water-point." When I get to the rock nobody was there! I looked around, yelled...nothing. I would have bet a check there was someone sitting there before! Continued on, and shortly after noticed a roll of Concertina Wire (razor wire) laying partially across the trail a couple hundred feet ahead of me. I remember thinking "That's a little dangerous, I will pull it out of the way when I get up to it."

Again...nothing was there."

While there is no hard and fast rules regarding hallucinations, your brain will generally replicate and exaggerate real people and themes from your immediate experience or imagination. Sometimes as with David these experiences are 'real' enough to fool you into interaction. In other cases things are bizarre enough that some part of your rational brain reminds you that you are sleep deprived and that what you are seeing likely isn't real.

More often than not however participants are persuaded by their exhausted minds into playing along with whatever show it wants to put on. Christopher Meredith experienced hallucinations of large groups of people during a near thirty hour endurance challenge at Ft. Bragg North Carolina:

"During Bragg Heavy 001 - on our final approach toward Dan's team house, I saw some amazing stuff! I saw little boys and girls running by our class on our right side (all in red shorts and blue shirts), off to the left side of the road, near a Semi, I saw a basketball team practicing (they were TALL too, LOL) and the best one was what I saw behind the team house, I think there was a hill there? I saw an entire picnic going on: BBQ grills smoking, kids with balloons running around, dogs chasing frisbees, and loads of people standing around. I remember turning to Eddie and saying something like, "Look, they are having a party for us as we finish out the first Heavy". That was a crazy day…"

These kinds of temporary blackouts (called 'micro sleeps') and hallucinations are worse at night. Your body is adapted to resting in times of natural darkness and so even when you are forcing yourself to stay active, your efforts will be markedly more difficult during hours of darkness. A few endurance challenges capitalize on this natural chink in our armor and host their events so that large periods of them will take place during the night. The night time also tends to make the woods and wilderness significantly more frightening to the primarily city dwelling population of these events. Dominique Gordon recounts the host of imaginary wildlife she encountered on her 24+ hour endurance challenge:

> "I thought I saw a bobcat during my Heavy. It was a stump. Someone in the group said , " Is that a bobcat?" All 13 members of my Heavy team were just staring , finally cadre said .. "It's a stump!!" Funny none of us were concerned that the bobcat would attack. Ha! Also, stepping on twigs became snakes, .. Oh a snake, hmmm. Ha ha."

Episodes during sleep deprivation can escalate when activity level dips which is one reason why you come across such fun stories from participants of endurance challenges where the activity level rollercoasters up and down as opposed to a continuous event like an IRONMAN. Any military veteran who has had to pull guard duty will tell you that staying awake while essentially sitting around can be a massive challenge. This can also happen (especially at night) if the task at hand is stationary and repetitive. With little to no new stimulus to keep you alert your brain will take every opportunity to shut down anything not being used. Avid endurance challenge athlete and CrossFit guru Jason Spare had an experience in just such conditions at one of the infamous Spartan Death Races:

> "During DR, about 48 hrs in, we were sequestered to an area to do hard labor. A woman near by felt sorry for us and cooked us burgers. In my sleep deprived paranoia, I climbed a tree to hide, convinced it was a trick to punish us more (I was clearly visible in the tree). They ate burgers, I sat like an ape in a tree for an hour. Then, there was that pig eating grass in the middle of the field that night.... There were no pigs."

New and novel terrain can add greatly to an athlete's stress and fatigue as they try to find the best way to deal with unfamiliar environmental variables on the fly. This includes hard to plan for factors like temperature differences, humidity, and altitude. The combination of these additional stressors will accelerate the coming of fatigue and its associated effects. Troy Gayer was hit by the increased fatigue and sleep deprivation as he trudged up the winding mountain woods and roads in Colorado during a customized 24+ hour endurance challenge:

"During NOGOA 001 (No One Gets Out Alive) when the team was on it's way back to the endex (End of Exercise), which was a long march that seemed never-ending, I fell asleep on my feet. I would still be walking forward in my column as I ran into the ruck in front of me. Bumping into that person would jolt me for an instant but two steps or so later I'd be right back to seemingly unconscious.

As for hallucinations, the light from our headlamps was casting shadows and every once in awhile mine would turn to look at me then run off ahead of me. Also, I kept seeing a Jeep stopping to pick people up, but then I'd walk through the back of the Jeep. Overall, it was a disturbing first experience with something I'd only ever previously heard of in books."

One of the enduring events in SFAS, other special unit selections, and GORUCK Selection is simply known as "The Long Walk". It is a rucksack march with an undisclosed distance and time standard. Suffice it to say it is long (hence the name) and it usually comes near the end of the event meaning that the candidate is almost completely spent going into it. This extremely long, monotonous event is when most candidates that make it that far have the most vivid and frequent hallucinations they will experience. Most of those Selected during GRS that I surveyed gave me a story from their Long Walk. So I put them all together here instead of trying to introduce them all individually. So keep in mind that each of these stories is from a different time and place and each participant was likely completely alone during the whole experience:

> "During Selection 008, on the long walk, I had quite a few hallucinations. I'm an auditory person, so at one point I could hear the lead cadre yell at me that there was water up ahead at certain point, but when I would arrive there, there was nothing there. I remember checking for his footprints on the side of the trail just to be sure he wasn't there. It must have been campers or loggers off in the woods, but my brain turned it into what I wanted to hear. I also saw a dragon during that walk, but that's another story" (John Maris).

"My worst hallucinations were at Winter Death Race in 2012. The Sunday morning "long walk" before dawn had me see a huge house party with music and lights in the middle of rural Vermont. It turned out to be a big tree in a field. I was convinced that this was the end of the Death Race with skull ceremony, and was really bummed out that it wasn't. I also saw a highway that we had to cross. No idea what caused that as there was nothing there at all.

During Selection 000 I hallucinated dolphins popping out of the water. I also saw toddlers running in and out of the surf and running around us as a group at one point. The other one was two fat naked gay guys holding hands walking along the beach at 2am. Turned out that one was actually real though" (Mark Webb).

"At Selection 000 I saw the tail lights of Chris's raptor for at least a couple hours during the long walk. In my mind it meant we were close to the end. Later during a break at maybe 4 or 5am we were sitting and I saw a woman in a bikini on the beach alone. I asked Greg "Who the hell comes out here this early?" He didn't know what I was talking about. I looked back and she was still there. But not really" (John Templeman).

"During Selection I was running before dawn on the second day. I went into a light trance state and "woke up" with a full head of visual memories that I hadn't ever experienced live. I can still remember it very clearly but it only exists as memories, I don't remember having actually been there. Like I saw it on TV" (Andy Capps).

"While on the night portion of our long walk, I would look into the ocean and see abnormally large shark fins and look up towards the dunes and see people hiding under the boardwalks. The swinging chem light in front of me on someone's ruck didn't help either. Kind of lulled me into a trance. Selection is horrible and should not be attempted by anyone" (Greg Stroud).

"I thought I saw Burt Reynolds (the Norm MacDonald spoof version) driving a yellow school bus in the second night of GRS 001. One of the many hallucinations that seemed so real. A long day's journey into night indeed" (David Kim).

The more time you spend in the endurance challenge world the more you will become familiar and sympathize with these stories as you cultivate your own. With proper rest and recovery such deprivations are temporary and will not lead to chronic states or major health deficits. While not fun at the time of the event, afterwards stories of your visions and mishaps will be hilarious barroom conversation with the friends you went through it with. These sorts of stories become like badges of honor representative of a sort of 'right of passage' to be able to share, and the understanding of how things are for frequent top level endurance challenge athletes.

Again everyone is different but snapping myself into focusing on others is my prefered method for getting out of a funk. When keeping to myself starts putting me to sleep and giving my body an excuse to succumb to fatigue I just bother other people. This is why the team leader is usually the most lucid member of a long running endurance event. Try it sometime, if you start droning just get yourself involved in someone else's business. Check their water, offer them food, ask them their mother's maiden name, that sort of thing.

Weathering the Storm of Doubt

"It's all in your head ladies and gentleman. When you show up for Selection you should look right at me and say to yourself, "I don't give a f**k what this guy makes me do, I will not QUIT, GFY". So when I am standing over you at the 48th hour and you're hating life, look up at me and smile." -Dan Plants

Being physically strong is not the only asset you will need to be successful when looking to tackle some of the harder endurance challenges on the market today. Mental toughness can be cultivated in a number of ways which often make for the best stories. For many, just training themselves physically in order to compete for a top spot in an event will require the forming of determination and mental focus. For others, life's experiences lend great poise and level headedness during times of duress (this is likely why many of the top finishers of the most grueling challenges are older adults with intense life experiences).

Harrison Lee Coale cultivated the determination and focus

he had accumulated over an entire childhood's worth of dreams and aspirations for military service. The urge to finish something once started is a strong one, especially when you are able to convince yourself that you started down a path decades ago and it is finally coming to fruition. For Coale this came to a head during a readiness event called the Texas Bug Out Drill. Bug out drills usually involve a little or no notice expulsion onto a long course of foot movement that is littered with both expected and unexpected challenges meant to be tackled with the gear you brought along in haste. It is a way of testing your resolve and your packing intelligence, for Coale he learned something about himself that was far more valuable:

Coale

I am currently a TACP candidate here at Hulman Field. When I was younger I woke up every day for four years wanting to join the US Military. When I was sixteen I went to an event in Texas called "The Texas Bug out Drill". It was a never ending hell for an out of shape sixteen year old. 10 miles into this event, a super cell rolled into the middle of the ranch where we were located and they canceled the event. However I had different ideas; my old man's military stories about never quitting had really stuck to me.

The director told me I couldn't leave the staging area, I told him where he could put that business and rucked off into the storm, much to the protest of the people running the event. Childish I know, but as I understood it at the time I had signed up for 15 miles. I had only done 10. I owed and I would pay my dues. It sheeted rained so hard nearly horizontally in the absolute most literal sense. I could not see my hand in front of my face. Tornado warning sirens sounded. A jeep came out, marked "Quitter Wagon" to collect me. I told them to piss off. They reported that there was: "A crazy guy who refused to get on the wagon." out in the storm completing obstacles.

My dad and an older mentor of mine just laughed, they knew who "The crazy guy" had to be. I met one other guy out in the storm, and we rucked the last five miles together; they were arguably the hardest five miles of my life. This was my first experience with understanding what someone is truly capable of. Pushing the limits of your endurance and willpower teaches you a lot about yourself, as everyone in this group undoubtedly knows. Since then, I've felt innately destined to have that be a part of my life. That day I decided that serving would be a part of my life as well.

No matter what happens, if you think you are supposed to do something, if you truly believe it is what you want to do, NEVER let anything or anyone dictate YOUR path. I think the reason people do things like this is to see if there actually is any external influence that could change your mind once you set your heart on the finish line.

The answer is no. -(Coale)

Once harnessed properly, determination can be a hell of an ally. I have often heard it said that determination and resolve is something that has to be learned through experience (and more often beaten into you), luckily as in Coale's case you can be the one to beat it into yourself if you are willing to take the risk. The task at hand doesn't have to be impressive to the world; even if no one else knows what you are doing, as long as finishing it is important to you.

Motivation for Current and Aspiring Endurance Challenge Athletes

You need to experiment and find out what drives you and can be the future source of your determination and resolve to succeed.

Motivation is a powerful tool in all aspects of life and can often be the only thing that gets one to start or finish a particularly challenging task or goal in life. Motivation can be internal or external and most people draw from some unique mixture of the two in their lives to 'get shit done' as the saying goes. Pride, vanity, conviction, friends, family, and loved ones have all been classical sources of motivation and all have the potential to be ultimately beneficial or negative for the individual in question in the long run.

Motivation can easily turn sour on you if you are getting it from the wrong place. Long term decisions made in states of high emotion and in fits of group think (often known as the ' visit from the good idea fairy' in the military) can seem idiotic and aimless with the sobering application of time and reality. Everyone is different and some people's half cocked plans turn out to be genius but in general planning ahead and taking time to meditate on what is truly important to you will reveal what is really worth working for. You not only want your accomplishments to materialize, but you also want them to be meaningful and deeply satisfying to you in the long run.

Motivation for Current and Aspiring Endurance Challenge Athletes

When you start examining these important things you will begin to realize what matters to you and where you draw your motivation from. If you are serious about endurance challenges then you will likely have to develop some kind of internal driving force unless you have a seriously intense purpose you are working for (and even then such conviction tends to develop internal motivation). That little voice in your head needs to be a positive one (and a resilient one at that) because when push comes to shove and you are beyond exhausted you are going to listen to that voice and if it wants to throw in the towel...chances are you will. Dana Lynn Whitmore gives us some insight into where her motivation to sign up for countless extreme challenges comes from:

> "I would say a good majority of it is internal. I like to push myself. I'm also lucky to have my brother, who without him I probably wouldn't have had the guts to sign up for my first GRC. I came across the event online, told him to check it out, and he texted me back 30 minutes later telling me he registered. So, I did too. I met my boyfriend during that first GRC, and it has been great to have him to train with and do

events with. We can do these things together and I think it helps to have a significant other that understands. My parents and other siblings root for us too, they live 1,000 miles away so training doesn't affect my relationship with them much, but knowing that they support what my brother and I are doing helps. My other brother and sister have become interested in doing one as well, so I'm hoping we can all 4 do one together as soon as the youngest turns 18!"

As we can glean from Dana's experience, motivation is both highly necessary and highly personal aspect to an athlete's being. There are so many potential sources for excitement whether it is from taking on the next personal challenge or repeating a completed event but with courageous and inspired friends and family in toe. Realizing what motivates you and harnessing it to augment your chances of success could easily be the difference between crossing the finish line and crawling to the medical tent with a lame excuse.

A word of motivation for female athletes looking to break into the world of endurance challenges (often still pegged as a 'guy thing' despite large numbers of female participants) from Dana Lynn Whitmore:

"I really do believe that you have to be a certain type of person to do one of these events. As a female, the notion that a GRC is a "guy thing" has actually never even crossed my mind (even though I've done 3 or 4 where I've been the only female). I think the important thing for them to realize is that a GRC is team based. If she is in the gym doing overhead presses with a dumbbell, I'd start comparing it to ruck presses in the event. Maybe start throwing in some of the things we do in the events into her workout routine so she knows she can do it. Squats with a sandbag, for example could mimic the weight she would feel doing squats with a ruck.

The GRL and the GRC are about having fun as well, and meeting new people. If you think about it, GORUCK is one big social get-together, and women LOVE get-togethers! After that, I think it comes down to heart, and personal convictions. Some people will just never do it even if they are perfectly capable. I think that's just fine. Everyone has their own goals in life, and if pushing themselves to see what they're made of, becoming part of an epic team, meeting awesome people, and doing something you will remember FOREVER, doesn't fit in with those goals, well...I don't think there's much anyone can say to convince them otherwise."

The dark side of motivated train up is of course burn out. It comes in many forms and can happen for various reasons but versions essentially mean a severe loss of interest in reaching previously set goals. Psychologists have long ago figured out that willpower is a finite resource that can be used up. Though like a muscle, natural athletes and those who work at it will accumulate larger reserves of willpower, the reserves are not infinite, and even the most seemingly dedicated athlete can become mentally exhausted, disillusioned, and generally fed up with training and events.

It is sometimes hard (from the outside) to discern whether

someone is mentally exhausted or if they are simply moving on to different priorities in their life so it is important to be supportive to the individual and help them 'wait it out' for a bit to see if they bounce back or if this change of pace is something they really want. The phrase 'sleep on it' holds a lot of wisdom and is applicable to numerous situations, this being one of them. Matt Ogle describes his situation with mild 'burnout' and how it is presenting in his life:

> "That's where I'm at now. I'm having trouble getting motivated for training, and with my date (for a major endurance challenge) a month out, that's bad news. I'm doing a challenge this Friday night with extra weight, and then running a half marathon on Sunday morning. So I'm going to see how I fare after this weekend, but I may end up pushing back my date if I don't feel great, or am having trouble getting after the training."

While in a perfect world an athlete would be able to ramp up to the hardest events by simply taking on progressively harder challenges until they reached their goals. The reality (especially for all us non-professional athletes) however is that all the other priorities in life make it so that we rarely get to progress at the pace that is ideal for us. Sometimes we try to jump too many steps and end up falling short. The learning experience and challenge is having the willpower to stay motivated, get back on the horse, and use what we learned to push even harder for our next attempt.

If you have the focus and drive to turn a failure into a positive learning experience you may just find that failing to finish your chosen event was in fact the best possible training experience you could have for your eventual successful attempt. Try some comparable events perhaps of slightly lesser difficulty and use your hindsight to fix your training and before you know it you'll be ready for another shot at your original goal. Jason Spare talks about some events he conquered in the wake of a missed finish that helped him toughen up mentally and better prepare him for his comeback:

> "This whole year with tougher challenges DR, Selection and SERE were dedicated to toughening up mentally. Selection, I wasn't ready, SERE: I faced cold water fears, DR: I proved I could go well beyond what I thought for >58 hrs. Putting myself in uncomfortable positions/places really helped toughen

me up mentally. Now, I need to complete these challenges. Also, the advice of doing a GR Heavy really helped it was a huge confidence booster that I needed, for I had doubts after Selection."

As you can tell there is no clear ranked list of events by degree of difficulty. Things are never that simple. Unfortunately even asking experienced individuals will only get you part way there as a group of people all having completed the same events will still rank them differently. The best thing you can do is do your homework and critically evaluate your personal abilities compared to the content of the event in question and try to come up with a battle strategy that way.

In events where you are on your own and even forced into isolation friends can be more of a liability than an asset. Especially in elite level events the dedication and drive required to succeed and do well is so high that in a circle of friends it is statistically very unlikely that they will all be able to rise to the occasion. Add to this the uncertainties of your personal situation and a lack of detailed information about what you are going to undertake (many events change things up and keep their challenges secret to prevent too much preparation) and you have a recipe for personal disaster.

Motivation for Current and Aspiring Endurance Challenge Athletes

Instead you need to focus on how much victory means to you personally. If the good feelings of success are only realizable amongst friends for you then you need to find an event that caters to that eventuality. Otherwise you need to make sure you are driven and focused enough to succeed on your own if necessary. Do your homework and prepare like your life depends on it. Robert Alban talks about the challenge he faced when preparing for GORUCK Selection in collusion with a number of friends and dealing with the reality of living in Germany and preparing for an event in Washington DC:

> "I read the AARs, anxiously awaited GRS updates, and finely combed through any GORUCK or third party YouTube/publication I could find. I was hooked on gathering information and preparing myself, yet still felt terribly unprepared. When it's hot outside and you're expecting snow on game day at an event that starts over 4200 miles from your home, it is hard to get and feel prepared. As the seasons changed, so unfortunately did the "commitment" of all but one of my crazy friends (and come the big day, he unfortunately didn't pass the PT test). Every day

GRS was on my mind, whether with specific training, logistics, or even theoretical debates."

Being able to push past the failure or non-commitment of those who came with you is a hard skill to cultivate and for some it takes all the flavor out of what they were looking to accomplish. This is something you need to find out for yourself and pick your events based on that knowledge. The great thing is that there are so many choices out there that finding events that fit your goals and ambitions is quite easy.

If you are part of a team looking to finish a long endurance challenge then you have a potentially valuable asset in your fellow team members. Emotions and doubts are like a rollercoaster ride with ups of self confidence and downs of crushing doubt and uncertainty. When on a team realize that each member is likely to be at a different point on this continuum at any given time. It is the responsibility of the members in the 'up' position to be the 'tough love' police for those in the 'down'. Reasoning with someone who is in a quitting mood is like talking to a drunk person, what they are saying might make sense but they potentially mean none of it and will regret subsequent consequences later.

In such instances I feel it is perfectly acceptable to take serious corrective actions on their part in order to keep them in the game until their mood 'swings back up' again. As long as they are not acutely injured, do what you have to do. Steal their car keys, throw their shoes into a river, dive tackle them as they trudge away, whatever it takes to keep them in the game. Believe me they will thank you for it when the event is over.

Just as keeping yourself focused on the task at hand and your priorities of work (feet, water, kit, food, rest) will help you continue on in your chosen event as an individual, keeping your team focused on the same is key to success. Use hindsight as a tool and don't make maintenance and refit plans that you know are unfeasible in a state of hunger, sleep deprivation, and near exhaustion. It is often best to forget anything fancy, keep things 'caveman' simple, and stay laser focused on the next task at hand whatever it may be.

Going back to succeeding as an individual, you have a lot to focus on which can turn out to be a bad thing. The human brain can only adequately quantify and evaluate so much at a time. This applies to time, mass, endeavors, you name it; if there is a whole lot of it then your brain will generally be pretty terrible at evaluating it. This means numbers become less meaningful as they increase and time ahead of you in an event becomes harder to grasp. This generally leads to mental chaos, and event organizers are counting on it. Signing up for a 48+ hour event is like climbing the ladder of the high dive, it is easy to click 'register' but it is way bigger once you 'get up there and look down' so to speak.

In a forty mile race it is counterproductive to think 'thirty eight miles to go' that outlook is going to cause you problems. The mind stays calmer and more collected when it has bite sized chunks it can easily handle. If the event has aid stations why not count them instead? Maybe set your watch (if you even bother to use one) to beep every five miles instead of one. In any case the saying "What is the best way to eat an elephant? ... One bite at a time." Is filled with wisdom for the endurance challenge community.

Most of what you need to stay focused on the increments of your race is mental control. Keeping yourself fueled and not letting yourself lag behind in calories or hydration will keep you sharp and rational (if you were either of those things to begin with that is). Unfortunately if your event does not allow calories or puts you out of reach of them you need to get some simple, effective mantras

drilled into your brain that you can recall even at your worst.

Most of the time you will be able to responsibly keep yourself fueled; this plus a good method of mentally parsing up the event will go a long way. This will be a constant process. Don't think that having a plan and staying fed will be enough, your mind will get bored and want to grasp at what you are doing big picture. You need to keep yourself focused either on the task directly at hand or on something far off in your imagination. If all else fails try and immerse your mind in something totally apart from what you are doing. Turn on your mental television and veg out as long as you can.

Selecting and Testing Your Equipment

Educating yourself on the elements involved in the event you have your sights set on and comparing that information with the variety of equipment choices available to you is a logical first step. But as is often said: experience is the best teacher. The hard truth is that unless you have comparable experience in closely related events or activities then you will never truly be able to account for all the possible variables involved as well as someone who does. Especially with physical events there is no better teacher than real world experience. So the hard reality is that in order to give yourself the best chance for success in your event then you are going to have to beat yourself up to the standard of your chosen endeavor.

Gear effectiveness and necessity tends to be a personal taste issue more so than other aspects of athletic events. While running would be considered universally necessary training for a marathon, what type of shoes to use will garner thirty different answers from thirty different first place finishers. This means that for the beginner it is important to be extremely skeptical with selection of equipment (especially if you are on a budget) and you may find it very helpful to find a store that is patient and accepting with testing their products out in store and has a very lenient return policy.

Do not abuse the system, as you will ruin it for the rest of us. However, there will be times when something you purchase will not work out as you expected and in that instance you will be thankful for being able to return the item rather than suffering through the lifetime of the product or worse, chucking it in the bottom of your closet never to be used again. Patience is a virtue, big box online retailers have great sales and excellent return policies so if you can wait for your gear to turn up there you can save a lot of money.

Asking advice from others is not a totally lost cause, rather it is always advisable to test recommendations to make sure the approach agrees with your personal style. Depending on the event you may get to know other participants who are of the same height, build, or athletic style as you and their advice may prove to be quite applicable to your style, but still a test is warranted. There may also be situations where the type of event would benefit from your team all utilizing the same equipment, in such a circumstance a middle ground should be found where the chosen gear fits all participants preferences as best as humanly possible.

Equipment required for peak performance at endurance

challenges can be a significant logistical and financial obstacle to would be participants. In some cases there can be a significant difference between required gear for participation (an official packing list that the event demands participants furnish for themselves) and optional equipment generally considered to be required for victory (what the winners are almost always using). This means that there can be a significant difference between what the baseline event costs and what someone looking to be competitive really needs to pony up.

All I can tell you is do your research and talk to as many successful past participants as possible. Scrutinizing the packing lists and learning the flexibility inherent in it along with a thorough analysis of the terrain and weather for the event will give you an idea of what additions and subtractions you can and can't make. Weight is another consideration. Is there a minimum weight? If not you should be scrimping and saving weight wherever possible, but if there is a minimum then you might be free to bring some useful gear without guilt.

I am not sure if it was the Army or something else but I immediately fixate on when a person makes up rules unintentionally.

When looking at a packing list, take it for what it says in exact english. Do not read extra context into anything, especially if it makes your life harder. For some reason there are athletes (mostly new but even some veterans fall prey) who either ask too many questions, or assume requirements that do not exist. For example: you would not believe the number of people I run into when working for GORUCK who assumed that they had to buy a special GORUCK backpack for the event even though event instruction never say such a thing.

I think I could do a whole book on this topic alone. To be brief here, realize that your event is run by humans not omnipotent deities. The packing list likely lists 'types' of items you will need and if there are pictures of the items you likely do not need to match brand and color. Also, many of these events are run by prior service military where they are used to obscenely specific and yet confusing packing lists. Unfortunately many of them will save themselves some keyboard time and just copy-paste and old military packing list for their event. So realize if you read: 'undershirt, individual, brown-dry fit, one each' on a packing list it means: 'bring a damn t-shirt'.

Now there is a very real difference between not being

intimidated by a packing list and coming unprepared. Realizing you can bring any damn brand of headlamp you can afford is not equivalent to "Meh it won't get that dark, I'm not bringing one." Required equipment is required equipment, as long as you have something that adequately performs that function you will be able to get by. But you will screw your team if you just leave things out to save weight or bother. If you ever feel tempted to leave a lot of things out just go watch Black Hawk Down, then come back and pack your bag.

I personally dislike what Alton Brown called 'unitaskers' meaning things that serve one purpose and one purpose only. For me this also applies to gear that I have no reasonable hope of using after the event. For instance I do not currently surf, dive, or snorkel so my buying a wetsuit for World's Toughest Mudder would have been a one off expense (an example of something that is not required or even mentioned but is generally considered to be mandatory by those serious about winning the event) and so I personally would look to borrow 'unitasker' items like this whenever possible or to buy them second hand in order to save yourself that well earned money. Christian Nelson shared a similar reality when preparing for World's Toughest as he describes:

> "World's Toughest is a large investment for someone like myself. I didn't own a wetsuit and I don't camp so I didn't own a tent or sleeping bag. I registered early, and then kept my eyes peeled for sales on wetsuits online. I ended up getting a great deal on a wetsuit from an online vendor. Borrow as much as possible; I borrowed a tent and sleeping bag from my neighbor and a friend was generous enough to cook for me and let me borrow thermoses for coffee and hot soups. WTM had to be in driving distance for me. I know a lot of people flew in for it, but being able to drive with the equipment was a necessity for me."

Equipment selection for events depends on the individual, and different athlete's choices for an event will range greatly between them. Some athletes will buy all new gear for different events while others will wear the same gear across events and until it literally falls off of them; Some pack more than needed in order to be prepared for variable situations while others pack as light as possible in order to save weight in exchange for comfort. While there is no right answer, preparation and experience are two constants when examining regular top finishers. Preparation includes mental, meaning that you should research every aspect of your chosen event to include picking the brains of previous finishers.

One of the learning games I always used to play after coming out of a field problem was to unpack my gear into two piles, one of things that I used, and the other of things I did not. This was to show myself what I had been carrying as pure weight, because I didn't use the gear, it was about as useful to me as a bag of sand of equivalent weight. For your events it can be helpful to perform such learning games after 'dress rehearsals' (training in the same kit you'll be competing in). One thing that I noticed in performing these self evaluations is that certain gear kept popping up in the 'used and useful' pile. I like to call this equipment my MVK (Most Valuable Kit) and more often than not it is the simple things that make the list. Matt Ogle elaborates on his approach to packing his gear:

> "I use a pack light philosophy for most events, and I like to experiment with new combinations so I don't really have anything that I use at every event. I also am worried about getting dependent on a piece of

gear, so I try to avoid using the same thing all the time. The closest thing I'd say to an every-event piece of gear that I have are Injinji socks. I love them."

The race and outdoor equipment industry is vast and varied, so much so that an athlete could get exceptionally good and experienced in a sport without ever trying or even hearing about all the equipment options available. The good news is that at even the most individualistic competitive events an athlete with even a sliver of social skills will have at least a few conversations with fellow athletes. And one of the most enduring and popular conversation topics is about gear.

Gathering excited recommendations from others about what to use during your next event is not the entire solution. Instead, it is a good place to start your personal experimentation in finding what works for you. Finding the best fit for you is quite a process, and having the positive reviews from your peers can help you navigate the jungle of high and low quality equipment out there. Individual experiences may vary so ask around and watch out for what I call the 'Yelp' reviewers who will rave about how awful a product is simply because the postal service (a factor unrelated to quality or performance) delivered their stuff late.

Michael Petrizzo has participated in some of the craziest CrossFit challenges I have ever heard of and is always one of the strongest members in any team I have been with him on. These types of challenges run the gamut of conditions and tests of strength many of which are for time which adds its own particular flavor of stress and self imposed intensity. All of these factors are incredibly hard on the body and in order to mitigate the potential damaging forces involved a successful athlete like Michael needs to select his equipment intelligently. Things need to work under any conditions, and hold up over time; here are some of his valuable recommendations:

> "From the feet up . . . Sportslick is a MUST. It is amazing. I only changed my socks 4 times during the Death Race and my feet were fine - hardly any wrinkling.

> Next, I'll never leave home without my Salomon Speedcross 3. They are, IMHO, the perfect multi-surface, multi-sport sneaker. They are super light, drain well, dry quickly, have an aggressive tread, and just the right amount of cushioning. I've

rucked with loads up to 100# on asphalt and my dogs never get hurt. They're GTG right out of the box. Oh yeah, they have a nifty Kevlar lacing system which comes in handy when my hands stop working from the cold.

For cold weather challenges, I looooove my Crye G3 Combat pants. They're expensive, but they are the GORUCK of pants. Light, customizable, allow for a ton of movement, dry well, and are tough as hell. They also have a ton of pockets for carrying food, sodium and gear.

For warmer challenges, Zioc Ether Mountain Bike shorts are the BOMB. Tough as all hell (quick repelling down a rope is not an issue), lightweight, and dry quick. Plus they have two zip pockets for stowing stuff, such as food and a sodium/ electrolytes.

Other than that, the only other must haves are my stainless steel leatherman multi tool, matches, and 50 feet of 550 cord."

Michael has been around the block enough times to have had some gear fail on him when he needed it most. Experience and hard testing have led him to trust and rely on these staples enough that he would recommend them, and that goes a long way. Again you need to take this advice in strides, the shape of your foot alone might make Speedcross 3's a terrible choice for you. But you can take it to the bank that recommendations from veteran athletes like Michael hold merit and that they are a good place to start when trying to find the best overall fit for your body and style.

More traditional endurance challenges like Marathons and Triathlons do not really require the athlete to continuously carry any sort of gear pack other than some micro storage for gels and water. However, there are a growing number of endurance challenges that either require a pack for added weight or simply by necessity because the event is so long. This adds a whole slew of additional variables to the athlete's physical preparations. Clothing choices, pack and carry options and of course what and how much to put into it.

One of the most important distinctions I have found that an athlete can make is the 'weight or packing list' distinction. This is easy to understand but all too frequently messed up by the uninitiated. When a required weight is stated, for instance GORUCK Selection requires you to have a pack that weighs a minimum of forty five pounds at all times without food or water, it actually benefits the athlete to have the heaviest/sturdiest pack possible. One simple source of discomfort when carrying a pack is too much weight in too small/unstructured of a pack. If you have to carry a bunch of weight then the best possible place to carry it is in the pack itself as opposed to the stuff that expands your pack ever outwards away from your back and center of gravity. A beefy external frame military style pack will be perfect in this case.

The other and more traditional possibility is that there are some required items (or items that you would be stupid to go without) but no specific weight. In this case you want to be as light as humanly possible. In general you will be weighing speed against comfort as the lightest packs also have the least support and padding, you will also be looking into the lightest weight high tech clothing to give you the protection you need for the least amount of weight. Just with these generalities it is easy to see the massive consideration and planning that an athlete needs to go through before they build the requisite experience to be able to 'intuit' these sorts of factors.

Another major factor is how you are built as an athlete. The fact is that when carrying things, smaller people will have to be more creative than larger ones. A small female athlete trying to take on a race with a large packing list can quickly find themselves with a pack that weighs almost as much as they do while the 6'3, 210lb athlete next to them is carrying only a fraction of their total body weight. Extreme endurance athlete and fit, petite female Hay Lee knows a thing or two about lugging massive packing lists and still staying competitive:

"I have always tried to think about packing as light as possible. Being barely triple digits in weight and 5'nothing, I attempt to level the playing fields when hanging with the big boys. But of course, I've always known that there are some essentials that can't be left behind, such as a mini First Aid kit. For my first GORUCK Challenge, I might have brought a bandaid and some super glue. For the Spartan Death Race, I packed about one of everything I thought I might need in order to save as much weight and space as possible, because you never know what that race will throw at you. A new staple to that "kit" would be salt tabs; I probably consumed about 25 over the course of the 75 hours of death racing. Electrolyte tabs have always been there, but I have since learned to bring more as it's just plain stupid to not continuously refill your water when allowed/available and be sure to have adequate electrolytes.

I'm always trying to think of ways that I can "double up" on certain items for the larger races. For example, I knew I would want something sharp, such as a needle, to pop blisters with. Well, why not simply bring a safety pin that can possibly have multiple uses?

When I first weighed my pack for DR, it was 65lbs (this would be 61% of my body weight). Minus the required gear, I had already thought over every item in my pack and wanted to keep it, except for my food. This might sound crazy to some, but I actually ended up taking out 95% of my "real" food (tuna, peppers, jerky, etc.) and solely packed a ton of protein powder and some tri powder (but that stuff is awful - I only used one pack). Besides being force fed a slice of pizza by a random support crew member around hour 58, (I had no crew of my own), the powder was my only "meals".

Team Wounded Wear Selection was about 16 hours and took place early February '13 during a cold front/storm in Virginia Beach. I had never participated in such a frigid challenge at that point. I did TONS of research on cold weather gear, as I grew up in the Caribbean, and my primary "cold weather" experiences were in Georgia. It was then that I learned the joy of hand warmers and dry socks. While only providing temporary relief, it's a small slice of heaven that can lift your spirits and convince you not to quit when you're feeling as low as I was.

For most of my challenges I have used a GORUCK Radio Ruck. While extremely durable and a timeless design, it's not the most functional or customizable (i.e. no waist belt, only 2 interior pockets, non-expandable, etc.). For the Death Race, I had ordered a Source Patrol 35L pack, which ended up being extremely too small with the surprise addition of 5 lbs of hay to the required gear list. I ended up borrowing a Mystery Ranch Crew Cab and fell in love. I did one training ruck with it before DR, but it was such a perfect fit and provided great comfort throughout most of the event. I will be looking to buy one in the future.

As far as packing for another Death Race, as of right now I would say that I will definitely be packing more moleskin and super glue. I had packed just enough for myself, but somehow what was left of my first aid kit around hour 60 was hijacked while I was off doing another event (sans ruck) - it definitely made the next 10 hours of racing slightly unbearable. More than anything though, it's your mental tenacity that will ultimately see you through to the end. But of course, it never hurts to have the appropriate, tried & true gear!"

When it comes to packs you have a massive number of options to choose from and unfortunately the only real way to figure out what is best for you is to test them out yourself. There are 'traditional' backpack bags with shoulder straps and a bag that generally has zippers and a variety of pocket configurations. These can be incredibly lightweight and packable but become very uncomfortable at weights over 25 lbs.

The world of real, weight bearing, 'packs' all have frames and a form of harness system. There are 'internal' and 'external' frames. Internal frames are generally favored by new high tech companies and are lighter and smaller than external, some companies will even custom mold harness straps for your body shape. External frame packs are the old standby of the military and can hold/secure massive amounts of weight and be very comfortable, the sacrifice you make is that they will almost always be heavier than internal frame packs (great for fixed weight events). In the professional climbing and hiking world there is a very good reason why any bag over 35L capacity almost always comes with a hip belt and chest strap. They make your life a lot easier and should be used whenever possible.

Packing your rucksack can be just as important as selecting it in the first place. Few things can be more frustrating and time wasting than tearing apart you pack because you didn't realize that the thing you packed all the way at the bottom was in fact the thing you were going to need often. For organizing your stuff you run into another trade off, packs that have tons of storage and accessory pockets tend towards the heavier side (when empty) while on the other hand minimalist packs require some creativity to prevent all your kit from becoming a big, cumbersome pile in the bottom of your bag.

Tricked out or minimalist you'll still need to analyse what you'll be doing and where you'll be doing it. If you know you are going to get wet then know that things in outside pockets are more vulnerable if not waterproofed. Things deep within your pack are more protected but if you are getting really soaked you will want to look into some sturdy dry bags to protect your stuff. For most events though you will get wet and muddy but no one will be diving or staying submerged for long periods of time. With this in mind there are a lot of high dollar waterproofing containers on the market. While these are great for Army Rangers, you will probably be better (and richer) off using an airtight freezer bag.

When arranging all the kit in your bag try and wargame out your event and use the scenario in your head (coupled with past experience if available) to figure out how to pack. Generally high importance or use items need to be easily accessible like your water source, quick snacks, and changes of socks. While less used items like sleeping bags or cooking equipment can be secured within the pack which is also a good thing because these items tend to be heavier and should be secured tight to the back and as high as possible.

As discussed before, when shopping for clothing and gear for your events there are a lot of options out there. Just like any other sport or hobby the price range for all the things you will need can vary wildly, and price is not always an indication of quality/characteristics you are looking for. Again, asking others is helpful in narrowing down your search (sometimes) but you will run into some big money weekend warriors who just walk into an REI and clean them out. These people have no issue paying full retail for stuff that "Looked cool", something that gives me heart palpitations.

A factor frequently overlooked by participants and particularly athletes coming to endurance challenges from other disciplines is the fact that you and your stuff is going to get beat up, scraped, muddy, and battered continuously throughout your event. With that in mind the Arcteryx wind shell for $499 retail starts looking like a bad idea. When I am in an event I want to focus on victory, not paranoia about scuffing up my new Patagonia pants I just blew half my paycheck on.

A savvy shopper with a little effort can find great deals from clearance websites (TheClymb.com and LeftLaneSports.com come readily to mind) and shopping the clearance sections on brand name sites. This method takes a little patience but can save you hundreds. Another oft overlooked resource that I take for granted living on military bases is the good old Army Surplus store.

Army Surplus equipment is usually cheap, comes in bland and easily cleaned colors and materials, and has generally been designed to take abuse. It may not always be as lightweight or as ergonomically laid out as brand name outdoor clothing but it will be tough and designed to work even in the hands of dirty, ham fisted neanderthals.

You would be surprised though at how many government contracts are picked up by brand name outdoor clothing companies. Arcteryx, Patagonia, Snugpak and more have products the Armed Services use that are essentially 'clones' of their much more expensive civilian doppelgangers. The only difference being that civilians are paying a lot more for interesting colors. A good example is the last pack the Marine Corp issued to its soldiers (ILBE) was designed by Arcteryx and was essentially the same as a pack retailing for nearly $500 (you can pick up an ILBE these days for around $70).

Knowledge is power, it may strike people as materialistic or over-concern with niggling details, but I believe that knowing the characteristics of the equipment and clothing you intend to use can only help you make the best choices. For clothing this generally means knowing how different types of fabrics react to the conditions present in your chosen event. Construction and design also plays a big part in determining what will give you the mobility you need to be as fast and light as possible without being miserable.

There is a reason why you generally don't see people show up to a Spartan Race in their favorite jeans and a t-shirt. In general natural fibers feel great, breathe, and hold up well. But in circumstances where you are moving fast and sweat, heat, water, and friction are involved, there can be some drawbacks. Cotton especially works against you when supersaturated (really really wet). This is because it can hold on to so much water that it gets very heavy and retains little body heat and takes a very long time to dry.

Wool has some great properties, it regulates body temperature, is tough, and retains a lot of your body heat even when soaking wet. It is however a heavy material and if layered incorrectly can speed overheating. The exception is a special performance blend made of Merino wool and other synthetic materials, products made from this performance blend are very popular right now and have produced some great results.

The Army used to make all its long underwear from a material called Polypropylene (Poly Pro in grunt slang), it is synthetic and quite warm. Amongst other reasons it was eventually ditched because it is quite vulnerable to UV radiation from the sun and does not wick moisture away from the skin as well as other products. It was replaced with a Polyester/Spandex blend that a huge amount of sport apparel is made out of today. This blend retains heat well, wicks moisture effectively, and dries in a reasonable amount of time. It is also stretchy and comfortable, just don't get caught in a fire with it on or you are in trouble.

The article of clothing that generally takes the greatest beating in these events is your pants. Finding a fabric type in a pair of pants you don't mind being seen in that can stand up to serious abuse can be a tall order, but there are plenty of options out there. Again cotton jeans are a poor choice for the same reasons we talked about before. And unless you are Pan or Lucky Ned Pepper you are unlikely to have fluffy wool pants.

One of the more tried and true fabrics you'll find out there is something in the range of a 60/40 Polyester/Cotton blend. This blend creates a tough fabric, and if it has a DWR (Durable Water Repellant) coating it can be quite weather resistant. One downside to this blend is that I have personally experienced a wildly varying range of quality and construction, with weight and durability fluctuating greatly from product to product.

Another potential downside to Poly/Cotton blends is that they can be heavy. Especially when soaking wet you can end up lugging around pants that weigh in at a couple of pounds even though they generally shrug off a lot of weather conditions and dry reasonably well. If you are looking into pants with this blend of material I highly recommend trying them on first (really you should do this whenever possible). The good news is that this blend of materials tends to be a little cheaper than others out there.

Cotton/Nylon and Nylon/Spandex blends are another popular choice and happen to be my personal favorite for endurance challenges. 100% Nylon is very tough, very light (or can be), and weather resistant. It's only drawback is that it isn't the greatest thing against your skin. It can get sticky or clingy when you are sweaty and rougher varieties will feel like sandpaper against your skin. For this reason it is usually blended with Cotton or Spandex to make it more 'skin friendly'.

Cotton/Nylon (usually a 50/50 mix) is very comfortable, lightweight, and durable. If you can get it in 'ripstop' it is even more durable. Nylon has a tendency to get lots of 'hanging threads', don't panic, your pants are not falling apart, just take a lighter to the threads and your problems are solved. This blend (NYCO ripstop for short) is what most modern military uniforms are made out of. The only downside is that with the comfort of Cotton you also get some of the negative water retention qualities and slow drying.

Nylon/Spandex (usually around 98/2 mix) can be VERY lightweight and tough. A good quality, well made set of pants in this mix is my go to for moderate to cold weather events, with a DWR finish wet and nasty weather will not be a concern for you. Drawbacks can be steep however if you select poorly. Some styles are loose and billowy like a tent and others can be tight fitting to the point where they stick uncomfortably to your skin. For this reason I like a medium weight tailored like regular pants with a low (like jeans) waistline as opposed to high (like dress pants) as these tend to be the sticky ones that are too tight. The Spandex is there because Nylon has no 'give' at all so make sure that the pants you select fit comfortably because they will never stretch.

The fabric combinations described above are generally concerning a 'traditional' choice in clothing as in underwear/compression shorts and 'pants'. However you are not limited to just this standard paradigm. Especially in colder weather you can experiment with all sorts of combinations of base layers and shells that have some interesting advantages and drawbacks that you may want to consider.

There is also a growing number of innovative outdoor clothing choices that incorporate hybrid fabric combinations to create unique and multifunctional pants and tops. While still quite expensive and produced by the more big ticket clothing companies this is likely where the future of technical clothing is headed. By combining different amounts of Nylon, Spandex, and Cotton and in strategically placed layers you will essentially have all the work done for you where making smart fabric choices is concerned. This technology will be especially advantageous in warmer temperatures where layering quickly becomes uncomfortable and even dangerous.

One company that does this hybridization particularly well is Kuhl. They make a lot of outdoor apparel but I am mostly talking about their pants. They make many many variations on essentially the same pant template. While not an insult (all the different types have different purposes) I will say that my wife (who is a badass but doesn't give a toss about pants) thinks they are all the same. But though the style is cloned the function is hard to beat in my opinion.

Most importantly for me (big smile here) they are big enough now to go on clearance at big box outdoor retailers.

I use their jeans now for everyday use because they rebel against the skinny jean trend, have a far superior pocket design, and have a little spandex added to make them incredibly comfortable. And while women figured out the spandex thing for their jeans a long time ago, the sewing and articulation Kuhl uses means I can do cleans and back squats in my garage gym without changing pants.

I also use many of their pants for expedition and endurance challenge events because they are tough enough but also comfortable enough to live in for a few days. Their convertible pants actually look like pants and many repeat endurance challenge athletes swear by them. I have recently started using a pair that is half Nylon and half Merino wool which means they are lightweight and retain warmth when wet. Another practical bonus for me working expedition events (in and out of the city and woods for a week at a stretch) is that Kuhl's look like real pants. Not looking tactical or homeless when you roll into town is nice for a change.

PrAna also makes some styles of pants made out of

seemingly magical fabric that is light, tough as nails, and normal looking. Again like with Kuhl's I believe this lies in product quality and construction as you can put them next to other pants of the same 'content' and be far superior. My advice from owning an embarrassing amount of outdoor clothing is be patient and frugal. Wait and watch for high quality, high function items to go on clearance and then scoop them up. In the end you will be happier than buying cheap crappy pants for convenience.

For ease of writing I will simply refer to any piece of clothing that is skin tight and worn next to your skin as a 'base layer' though that is technically not correct. The market for base layers is immense and ranges from true base layers that are designed to go against your skin and be worn under other articles of clothing, to pieces that are designed to be worn on their own. Many of these base layers have varying properties but in the caveman/woman world of endurance challenges they end up functioning somewhat similarly.

Your standard, entry level base layer is going to be

made of a mixture of Polyester and Spandex, the former for warmth with light weight and moisture wicking properties, and the latter for stretch and comfort. These base layers are quite affordable and function just fine, they do tend to be a little irritating against the skin over long periods of time especially during rigorous activity (it will pull chest and leg hairs) but this is only minor and the whole thing controls moisture and dries quite quickly.

Compression garments are what I would consider to be the next step up from the basic base layer. My personal go to favorite, compression layers improve blood circulation, reduce muscle fatigue, support joints and ligaments, and in some of the nicer brands help regulate body temperature. Compression layers are not just universally tight but instead utilize a variety of fabrics to 'squeeze' certain areas to provide support. Think of a sports bra for your knees, elbows, hips, and back.

Compression layers will also be primarily complex combinations of Lycra, Spandex, and Polyester. Some people love them and some not so much but the science behind their functionality is very solid and the nicer brands are very well made and durable. You get what you pay for here, and in general I have found that the nicer brands really do produce a generally superior product. Another fringe advantage of compression garments is that many of them are designed to be worn as 'stand alone' clothing especially if you are just going on training runs/swims and not rubbing yourself against rocks or concrete.

An addendum I want to include here is that time is a factor with compression garments and it effects my wearing them for an event. I am a white Scandinavian male so we may not have the same skin issues but in my case it is sensitive. For a strict race like an ultra run or a flavor of triathlon I still would reach for compression but when things get longer than twelve hours and especially when dirt, mud, and grit get introduced that time limit plummets.

Compression garments are necessarily very tight to your skin. This creates pressure which increases blood flow and prevents it from pooling. This is great when worn as a stand alone layer (and to their credit many compression company's recommend this as the only use) but when layered under pants the reduced airflow builds heat and clogs pores. This can lead to some really nasty business in the crotch region. Especially if any foreign matter gets in there it will be mashed into your skin. In the same manner anti chafing products can actually backfire and just act like smearing bacon grease on a teenage boy's face.

A shorter endurance challenge like a Spartan Sprint or if I was shooting to set a Tough Mudder time trial personal best I would likely go with compression still. However, for filthy events longer than twelve hours I leave the compression at home. The drawbacks just end up outweighing the benefits. Living in a full compression suit for essentially an entire day is no fun.

The fifty something hours I spent in my CW-X (which I love) suit at GORUCK Selection were horrible and the nightmare crotch scenario before my eyes as I peeled them off almost made me cry in the shower. Then again I used the same suit for a ten mile and then a forty mile mountain trail race in 2015 and loved it. In other words, if the event is fast and clean then I highly recommend compression garments.

A natural and yet quite high tech alternative is Merino wool base layers. This material is a unique wool that is comfortable enough to be worn next to the skin. It dries admirably fast but its real strength is that it loses little heat retaining ability even when soaking wet. Merino wool's main selling point is that it is one of the leading materials in regulating body temperature (keeping you cool when it's warm and warm when it's cold), Being that it is a natural fiber it has a distinct advantage in this category.

It is also favored by the military for tankers and pilots because when mixed with NOMEX it makes a garment that is quite fire resistant (synthetic materials generally turn you into a human Napalm torch if exposed to flame). Merino wool is a pricey material and the tailoring to make a high quality base layer garment out of it isn't cheap either. For this reason Merino wool base layers tend to be one of the higher cost choices out there but they tend to be worth it in terms of fit and function.

One mistake that I often see participants making with their clothing choice for an event is just wearing their favorite base layer garment as a stand alone piece. If you are just running or even swimming then this can be a perfectly acceptable thing to do; however, during an endurance challenge this is a bad idea. They are called base layers for a reason. They on average have little in the way of toughness or abrasion resistance. Pants and shirts, and especially the active and outdoor variety are designed and treated to be tougher and more abrasion resistant than the fabric normally is.

Base layers do not receive this treatment as they are designed to be thin and breathable when worn under other clothing. Wearing them alone is a sure fire way to tear holes and gashes into your new Merino top. In addition a lot of their beneficial properties become compromised when slathered in prodigious amounts of mud, dust, and dirt. Best to just keep them under other clothing.

The world of jackets can be just as complex as other clothing options and with higher price tags to boot. To be overly general the bulk of jackets you run into in the outdoor industry will fall into one of four categories: Fleece, soft shell, wind shell, and hard shell. There are plenty of new options out there that combine characteristics of two or more of the aforementioned categories and continuously evolving technology makes the downsides of these choices smaller and smaller. However, as always I like to sympathize with the athlete on a budget and the 'run of the mill' garments in these categories will generally fit the stereotypes I am going to describe.

Fleeces are for keeping warm, they can be microfiber or shaggier materials but their primary goal is to be soft, comfortable, and warm. Fleeces are great for wearing in calm conditions where you don't expect a lot of environmental adversity. This is the opposite of endurance challenges and so except for as a layering garment in extremely cold and slower events, you generally do not see a lot of fleeces during the race (before and after absolutely). In anything other than Summer time I throw a fleece in my change of clothes bag because they are lightweight and comfortable.

The thicker the fleece the heavier and harder to pack it is. This means that a fleece you can pack away and won't weigh you down when on the move is going to be lighter and necessarily somewhat less warm. In general, the lighter a fleece is the less wind and water resistant it will be. That said, the main drawback of fleeces is that they are not generally wind or water resistant to any meaningful degree, wind cuts through the breathable fabric and it soaks up water like a sponge. Modern synthetic fleeces do however have quite impressive heat retention when wet.

Next up is the more high tech and cutting edge soft shell. There used to be no category between fleece and hard shell and regulating your weather resistance and warmth came from layering and donning and doffing different combinations of these layers. The soft shell was developed in order to give a better option for multiple circumstances, especially where spending a lot of time adjusting layers was not feasible or safe. Soft shells are weather resistant enough to deal with wind and light to moderate rain while still retaining breathability and quick drying properties.

Soft shells are one of those clothing categories where you get what you pay for. The technology is not that simple and it takes quality construction and composition to make a great soft shell. So shop around and remember that it is designed to do the job of two jackets and so costs more. If you have the money for a good soft shell this is probably my highest recommendation for a good endurance challenge jacket.

With a soft shell you will need to change layers less and yet still be protected from a lot of the elements you will face. Of course it won't protect you from front flipping into a freezing lake and if you cake anything in enough mud it generally stops doing what it was designed to do. With that in mind though it is a great category to explore.

Hard shells are a pretty big category as they simply mean any jacket that is designed to completely keep water and wind out. This can be accomplished in a number of ways but of course the most modern are going to be the lightest, most flexible, and most expensive. Old school 'hard shells' can even be canvas coats with a heavy wax coating.

The advantage you get here is unparalleled weather resistance but at the cost of reduced ventilation and in some cases restricted movement.

If looking for a hard shell for an endurance challenge I would highly recommend browsing the sport of alpine mountaineering. Everything in that world is lightweight, packable, and in the latest and greatest cases even quite breathable with certain augmentations and extremely high tech fabric. I would advise against a big clunky hunting jacket as they are designed for sitting in tree stands for hours, not sprinting over obstacles and doing burpees.

If you are looking for a hard shell for endurance challenges I would suggest looking for something with plenty of vents that zip open, this way, during intense exercise you won't be doused in sweat trapped inside the jacket. Also make sure that when you are turtled up (zipped up with the hood up and cinched down) you can still perform basic human functions and have some sort of field of view. One of the major downsides to hard shells is that unless you are getting top of the line models they tend to take up space and be heavier than fleeces. The nature of the fabric treatment tends to make them hard to pack down.

One note I want to make about all three of these categories is how important their 'hardware' is. Hardware is a slang term for buttons, zippers, shock cord, flaps and snaps. Any method for closing up or securing the pants or jacket in question will likely be the weakest link on that piece of equipment and the most likely part of it to fail in adverse conditions. Remember when shopping that the warm toasty outdoor store is not the place you ultimately intend to use the product and so gives you a false sense of the product's durability.

My rating here is subjective of course but I would challenge almost anyone to find a better test of fastener than being dragged through the Quikrete like clay of Ft. Bragg for 24hrs with little to no fresh pond water baths. That said, I find simple to be best. Ties (like shoe laces) will generally function as long as you can get your knot out, with lashing straps to be a close second though few if any garments use lashing straps (almost exclusively found on packs).

Buttons with eyelets work almost all the time as long as they are well sewn. Zippers need to be of the highest quality to be of any use in these muddy, gross situations. In general the bigger the zippers the better, the main downfall of alpine mountaineering jackets is companies use tiny zippers to shed weight not anticipating that you are going to be caked in clay. Metal snaps are probably the worst form of fastener to use in these sorts of events as even a small amount of debris in the snap will make it likely to fail. Velcro is another contender for bottom position. Not only does hook/loop fastener perform poorly in muddy conditions, but it also has significantly shorter useful life span than the other hardware listed.

Another aspect that applies to both clothing and packs that is often overlooked is drainage. Whether there is a mandatory minimum weight or simply a packing list of essential equipment you don't want to be carrying any additional weight around. This is especially true if that extra weight is salt water and mud/sand. It seems trivial but water and earth weigh more than you might think. Having your bag

and cargo pockets stuffed with it will take a toll on you

quickly, all the while caking and destroying whatever it

shares that pocket/pack with.

Commonly called 'grommets' or 'drain holes', these

fixtures are common in military packs but less so in the

civilian market. They simply allow any water or fluid to drain

out of the pocket or compartment they are fitted to where it

would otherwise be trapped depending on how water

resistant the pack material is (unfortunately a material that is

great at keeping water out is usually just as good at keeping

it in). While you may have to go looking for a specialized

military surplus store or wilderness outfitter it is not

impossible to get these drain holes added to a pack you

already have.

Drain holes are even less common in clothing

(mostly pants are what we are worried about here).

However there are some smarter solutions that have been

devised for this issue. I am a huge fan of cargo pockets in

most circumstances but they have to be well constructed

and thought out to prevent them from being a hinderance to you during an endurance challenge. A traditional cargo pocket (large rectangular pocket on side of leg) needs to have a well secured flap and preferably some way for water to drain out.

Rocks and sand can be scooped out by hand which is actually the disadvantage of some of those artistically designed pockets in newer hiking pants (apparently thought up by designers bored by rectangles) because they are not big enough for your hand to 'scoop' anything out and many modern pockets do not 'turn out' in order to save weight on material. However, a smart aspect of these newer designs is that in order to make the pants more breathable the pockets are now a highly durable mesh inside that also lets water rush out very quickly and efficiently.

When considering events with multiple sections a lot of critical thought and planning needs to go into the down time between legs. In general these recovery times are misplanned in one of two opposing ways. Either little to no planning has been put into recovery and resupply. Or participants bring so much stuff that a majority of their time is spent trying to find things and make equipment decisions. With a little forethought and common sense drifting into one of these two extremes becomes far more preventable.

Advice and strategy in the context of an actual event might be better than generalized maxims. I will use GORUCK's HCLS as it is an event I have personally completed. It covers a wide spectrum of physical strength and endurance disciplines, and it is very long at fifty hours with three short breaks. This combination of factors makes for an approach strategy that is big enough and multifaceted that the reader can pick apart aspects that will apply to their chosen event and those that don't. This newer type of event will be covered more in the next volume of this series. But in the mean time see Chris Holt's detailed account of GORUCK's HCLS in the 'Some Extra Stories' section entitled: 'Back to Back to Back to Back Endurance Challenges.'

Motivation for Current and Aspiring Endurance Challenge Athletes

Active Recovery and Intelligent Event Approach

With the mentioning of body maintenance comes the inevitable discussion of recovery. There is no question that today's most extreme endurance challenges place intense stresses on the body and mind. Though the human body has an amazing ability to brace itself against stress and regenerate, the grind sustained from the abuse we put it through will break it if taken too far. Recovery is an integral part of an athlete's training program; those who ignore it will not find themselves highly competitive for long. In both training and competition failure to allot recovery time to yourself will likely result in plateaus and recurring pain/injuries.

What a lot of first time endurance challenge takers do not count on however is the mental side to recovery. Because these challenges tend to revolve around singular events there is the potential for an athlete to dump all their expectations and motivation into a single focal point. While this might make them extremely dedicated it also puts them at risk for some interesting and unpleasant feelings post event. Endurance athlete Dana Lynn Whitmore explains her initial tactics for physical recovery when her first Goruck Heavy (24+ hour endurance challenge) class 001 at Ft. Bragg North Carolina ended. She also talks about the unexpected mental challenges posed by the sudden loss of a training focal point:

"I've experienced two different sides of the recovery. I didn't really have a plan after Bragg. That was the first time I have ever done anything over 12 hours. What happened was a disaster. I caught up on calories, and rested, but I also felt somewhat depressed after. It was like I had been training for that for so long, now it was over. What do I do now? I ended up not doing anything for two weeks. I had a plan after my next one; I rested, caught up on calories and hydration, foam rolled/stretched and I was back to my normal activities on Tuesday. I definitely recommend going into these events with a recovery plan."

It is entirely possible that you are intending to train up for and execute your endurance challenge with no intention of any follow on events. This tends not to be the resulting reality as people tend to develop an affinity for particular events especially if there are more difficult 'rungs on the ladder' still left to climb so to speak. However, if the event concludes and after catching your breath you smile and decide to walk away with your finisher's prize and never return to the world of endurance sports then more power to you and make sure you follow a comprehensive and medically sound physical recovery plan to ensure that you will return to daily life no worse for wear.

Recovery can be like flossing, it is extremely hard to start and even harder to continue doing regularly. Yoga, Pilates, and good old stretching can be seen as a waste of precious gym time and slower (read: boring) pace that high intensity athletes find oppressively time consuming. Mobility, posture, and flexibility are too often ignored for these and other reasons which unfortunately leads to high numbers of injuries in high intensity athletic circles. What is important to focus on is the reality that an hour here and there stretching, resting, and breathing is potentially preventing you from going through the torment of six to eight weeks of rehab and recovery from a torn ligament or tendon.

Stretching, rest, and nutrition are the athlete's insurance policy. While certain causes of injury do not care about how much you stretch, there are a vast number of careless abuse and overuse injuries that a little tender loving care can go a long way in preventing. With a wide variety of styles of stretching, yoga, and pilates out there to chose from only the most stubborn athlete will fail to find something they can submit to once or twice a week. Also with the general minimalism of equipment used in such disciplines, a crafty athlete can reap the benefits of these disciplines without purchasing costly packages or having to attend multiple gyms.

Though the name recovery has an air of post-event activity it also applies to the time immediately prior to the event as well. A mistake often made by athletes is not taking adequate time to let their bodies recover from the intense train up before the start of the event they were preparing for. This means adequate sleep and nutrition as well as mobility and stretching activities. Endurance athlete Hay Lee discusses her personal struggle with pre and post event recovery and how she works to integrate it into her routines.

"Ahh recovery... my nemesis. An issue I'm finally starting to pay attention to after my first severely painful crossfit workout a few weeks ago. I've been "sucking it up" dealing with my shin splints for 9 months until the pain almost took me to tears during my workout. So, I went to an amazing PT as a recommendation from a fellow, local GRT (GORUCK Challenge finisher). I was left exhausted for days and with bruises for weeks - but he alleviated most of my aches - and discovered a ton that I never knew I had. I've since started listening to my body more and after my Spartan Beast this weekend, I'll be taking a "winter hiatus" from racing and attempting to focus more on R & R after hard workouts."

"The week leading up to a race, I will attempt to get more sleep than usual (which I average 5 hours/night) but that never happens. I'm a huge procrastinator and always end up staying up the entire night before packing and over thinking what to bring (at least for the bigger races). I typically go into an event having been awake at least 20 hours already, or at least gotten only a couple hours of sleep the night before. One might think that's insane, but I actually feel it helps me "get in the zone" quicker. I'm not a morning person anyway... it takes me a while to get "warmed up"!

I do start intaking Chia usually a few days before a race - I'll throw it in yogurt or oatmeal, and usually have a water bottle of it the hours leading up to the race start. I usually reserve the Epsom soaks for post-race, and only if I'm extra achy or have open wounds. For some reason, I actually loathe stretching, icing, etc. I know I should do it, I just never think about it and when I rarely do, I don't feel like doing it. The months leading up to Death Race, I actually bought a few hot yoga packages to force myself to go about once a week.

I HATED, I mean H A T E D it - the most extreme discomfort I had ever experienced... but I feel it aided dramatically with recovery from the slight aches and pains I had due to crossfit, etc. and also assisted in dealing (mentally) with difficult moments during DR. After DR, I went to regular yoga a few times merely for the stretch factor, but currently it's nonexistent in my life. I might currently stretch or foam roll for a total of 10 minutes/week."

Stretching can be like flossing for many (hard to start and easy to quit). There is just too much evidence out there today pointing towards active recovery being beneficial for an athlete to ignore this sort of TLC though. Disciplines like Yoga can often be a middle ground for some athletes who habitually put off stretching because they are crunched for time and want to get a workout in. By pushing your natural range of motion and flexibility you can get a great stretch in and feel like you still came out of it with a productive workout.

There are some other recovery techniques outside of simple stretching that an athlete can utilize before, during, and after their event. Especially when endurance challenges are taken on regularly, speedy recovery becomes a top priority to keep you in the game. To this end it can be beneficial to approach recovery from multiple angles (a whole body approach). A plan that includes rest, range of motion techniques, focused nutrition, and comfort activities can be a fast track to your next challenge. Not to mention that finding a recovery plan that works well for you makes you feel good and therefore makes the overall journey more enjoyable. Remember that having fun is one of the reasons you got into all of this in the first place!

First off is rest, it is the original and still reigning champion of recovery techniques. It is the simplest thing in the world and so the easiest one to ignore. Some resources out there like "www.sleeplikethedead.com" can help you figure out how to improve the quality of the sleep you are getting, but the bottom line is that you need to get some. It is the best way to 'hit the reset button', bring back your mental acuity, and repair damaged muscle tissue naturally.

Working on range of motion is sort of a catch all term for some of the flexibility techniques we have talked about previously. The bottom line is that you should find something you can tolerate on a regular basis or even better actively enjoy doing as part of your training routine. Yoga, Tai Chi, myofascial release, or even a stretching video from a commercial fitness collection are all at least starting blocks for keeping yourself injury free and in the game.

Focused nutrition is immensely important for anyone trying to compete for top spots in any athletic event. This is going to take some reading and research as much of the techniques are not perfectly intuitive but it is well worth your time and attention. Learn how to properly eat and hydrate before your event. Depending on what sort of event it is this could vary widely. Eating during your event largely depends on how much you can carry, whether or not you get to stop and rummage through food bags, and the consistent intensity levels you will be hitting during the event.

Maltodextrin supplements can be versatile for a variety of events as they can usually be mixed into water bottles or bladders or can be mixed thick into a facsimile of gels and Gu's for a fraction of the price. Electrolyte supplementation is also important; many powders claim to provide both easily digestible carbohydrates and electrolytes but make sure before you buy. In my experience I find better quality ingredients and more options if I keep my carbohydrate and electrolytes separate (I usually use a powder for the former and a capsule for the latter). Again, you will want to test all of this in your training to see what sits well with your stomach and mechanical preferences.

Eating for recovery is also very important for getting you back in the game and on your training regiment. Immediately following your event it is important to eat to regain your glycogen stores and begin to rebuild muscle tissue. Afterwards though you can go back to a more natural and healthful diet high in the proteins needed for repair and low in the carbohydrates that spike insulin at low intensities and hinder performance. I have not mentioned hydration because it is too simple. Drink water, millions of years of human hydration has not been improved on and there are no short cuts here, drink water.

To clarify that last sentence most sport drinks are garbage. The worst of them are detrimental and should be ditched for water. The best of them can help but come with a price tag (Kill Cliff cost more than a gallon of gasoline). Again the inconvenient truth involves work...make your own. This way you'll know what is in it and you will avoid the garbage big companies cram into sports drinks to drive down the price.

Making your own supplements is the only cost effective way to control what goes in your body. All it costs is that little thing we talked about earlier… time. Most sports drinks are sweetened with sugar to be cheap or corn syrup to be cheaper. Both sweeteners contain a lot of fructose which is a poison at rest and surely not something you want to be pumping in when going all out. Here's more bad news:

'natural' sports drinks like to use things like Agave syrup or brown rice which are even higher in fructose than simple table sugar.

What your muscles run on is glucose, it works but it is more expensive. With a little effort you can find pure glucose syrup and mix it into water at any percentage you choose. Today my endurance challenge 'go to' go-go juice is a mixture of lemon juice, glucose syrup, and Morton Lite salt. Table salt is all sodium, but Morton makes a 'lite' salt that is almost 50/50 sodium and potassium AKA electrolytes. I have personally seen great improvements in my mental acuity and general well being during events after switching to this approach.

Comfort activities are the carrot at the end of the stick. This term is deliberately vague and pretty much means any activity that soothes and relaxes you without hindering future endeavours. Soaking in an epsom salts bath or hot Yoga could be lumped into this category. This could also be as simple as taking a training day off and going for a nice sunny walk or take a long relaxing sit in the

Motivation for Current and Aspiring Endurance Challenge Athletes

hot tub, whatever floats your boat. Just make sure it is

something that lifts your spirits and can help you 'reset' and

be ready to go back to the grind working to attack that next

event.

Nutrition

Food is fuel for life and what you decide to put in your mouth can contribute greatly to your performance and well-being before, during, and after any event. As with any aspect of health and fitness the field is multifaceted, involving many moving parts which prevents the kind of 'miracle pill' or 'one step solution' that the diet food industry thrives on. For that reason the advice, stories, and recommendations that you read in this section may not always sync up and in some cases might be contradictory.

To that end, few of the athletes that the following information was garnered from are professional nutritionists and should not be treated as such. What they are though, are seasoned and successful athletes who have tested, approved, and rejected a number of dietary approaches and techniques. This accumulated social wisdom is worth examining if for nothing else than indicating the direction of the correct answers and warning away from easily made misconceptions or reasoning errors.

Motivation for Current and Aspiring Endurance Challenge Athletes

KISS

Nutrition is a huge portion of the active lifestyle and this goes double for people looking to be competitive in high performance events. This doesn't necessarily mean that there needs to be massive meal planning before events though. If you already engage in a lifestyle that centers on eating and performing well then only slight tweaks need to be made pre and post event. Nutrition is not a bandage or an energy supplement that can help you out in a pinch. To be truly effective you have to be making the right dietary choices as part of your everyday life, not the week before an event. Christian Nelson talks about his regular habits, his tweaks, and his silly rituals, note how all of it revolves around a massive lifestyle change that is now his everyday reality which gives him a great base from which to perform:

> "I tend to eat pretty healthy most of the time. I'm terrified of getting fat again so I tend to stick to a slightly modified paleo diet. I'm about 90% paleo. Tough Mudders, I don't really do anything different, I just try to hydrate if it's going to be warm. GRCs I try

to eat a meal a couple hours beforehand. One of my challenges I did I had a Buffalo Chicken Sandwich and I felt great the entire challenge. I never felt the urge to eat again. So it's a bit of a superstition for me, but if I can do that before challenges now, I do."

What you are not hearing about is some kind of juice cleanse or herbal supplementation being the key to Christian's success. The simple statement "I tend to eat healthy most of the time" implies a whole lot of corners not being cut and a harder road to travel than most Americans today are willing to venture down. Steamed fish and vegetables cooked in grass fed butter seems too simple to be ignored but you would be amazed at how many people know that this is more of the sort of thing that they should be eating and just aren't doing it. It is the worst kept secret that no one takes advantage of.

Keeping a clean nutritional lifestyle like this provides a base that takes a lot of the work out of event preparation. For less extreme events this can mean as little as a few extra servings of complex carbohydrates and an extra glass of water a few hours before game time. It also means that you and your friends can splurge on a little victory meal post wrap up per Christian's ritual: "Post challenges we have a bit of a ritual like a reward dinner. We just eat whatever we feel like. Pasta, ice cream, cheesecake, whatever. It's probably not the smartest thing, but it's what I do." By that point you are just replenishing depleted energy stores, and by picking up where you left off the next day you will hardly miss a beat.

The above is an example of why looking at nutritional choices as a lifelong process and commitment is far more versatile than as a diet focused on a specific goal. Realizing that food is for nourishing your body and fueling it for life's challenges allows you to sensibly modify your intake to best meet your goals. Approaching eating from the strictures of a set diet plan often restricts people from trying new things or exploring their possibilities for fear of violating the 'rules'. Even worse is when people attempt to take on intense physical challenges while sticking to their overly restrictive diet plans. Often this simply results in a failure to complete or meet personal goals. In the worst cases it can also lead to severe health hazards and medical emergencies if people ignore their bodies and try to push on regardless.

One of the major issues with all 'diets' (a misused word to begin with) is their overly restrictive nature as stated above. Another side effect of continuously restricting yourself is that your brain is too smart for that sort of thing and will end up stabbing you in the back by setting 'finish lines' after which you can relax and inevitably gain back all the weight lost. This is commonly called the 'diet treadmill' and for good reason, you can do it forever and you never seem to get anywhere.

Now during all of the above nonsense when do you have time to train? Where will you get the energy? The answer is never and nowhere respectively. Why do you think that one of the most common responses a bodybuilder will give to the question of "How do I get bigger?" is "Eat more, and lift heavier stuff more often." Food is meant to be fuel and without good quality calories, and lots of them you will have a miserable and largely unsuccessful time of training for your event.

If you don't believe me go try to have an upbeat conversation with a bodybuilder when they are 'cutting' for show season. If you don't get punched in the face you will likely get terse and impatient responses. Why? In order to compete bodybuilders need to eliminate every tiny bit of body fat and water weight to get their physiques to 'look' in top form. This means they are calorie deprived and dehydrated which takes huge amounts of willpower and focus. This is possible for them because it is not what they do most of the time and it will come to an end after show season. Their diets are similar to high grade versions of commercial weight loss programs. Sound sustainable for a lifetime? Hell no.

Will power as we will discuss later is a finite resource that can be worked out like a muscle but ultimately runs out and needs to be relaxed and recharged. If you are exhausting all your willpower on your crazy crash diet you will have nothing left over for your daily life and especially physical training schedule. The idea is to do your research and find a nutritional plan that fits your personal needs and satisfies you the right way. Such a nutritional lifestyle will use up little or none of your willpower reserve (if not boosting it greatly) leaving you free to crush it in the gym every workout.

So what should you eat as part of a healthy, sustainable nutritional regimen that will give you ample energy and satisfaction in your athletic lifestyle? That is not just a different book, it is a whole series of different books. You need to ask questions and do your own research. If doing that sounds like a pain in the butt and a lot of time just remember how much you eat in a lifetime and the effects eating has on the people you see every day. open your eyes to that and you will start to understand that this is a subject worth spending some time and energy on.

Every athlete I have met has different eating habits and preferences. However there are some similarities that are common. Eating simple and fresh food is one of them. The best explanation I have run into for the generic 'fresh, simple food' uses the modern day supermarket as a template. *Cook This Not That!* by David Zinczenko gives the simple advice to "Stick to the outside of the store." This is where you find the produce, refrigerated sections, and deli's. Foods in these areas generally have fewer ingredients, less processing, and less preservatives.

This is personal advice but I have found that cooking for myself has not only been great for my health and training but just plain great as far as life skills go. Home economics was demonized so much during my middle and high school days that I would wager that most of my graduating class has no idea what to do with fresh produce. They certainly do not know how to turn it into food. So my advice to starting a healthy athletic career is learn to cook for yourself and your family and take the time to learn about food in general.

So lets say that you have your healthy lifestyle all figured out and you've been living this way for long enough to have energy left over to train up for some endurance challenges of your choosing. What do you pack for the event? Ahh, now here is an area fit for this book. There are serious pro's and con's to any kind of food or drink you try to bring along to your chosen event with numerous factors weighing in. Here, with the help of experienced endurance athletes, we will explore what works, what doesn't work, and other many and various lessons learned that can help you avoid falling back on trial and error.

One aspect to race day nutrition that is often overlooked even by the experienced is the issue of access. You need to do your homework and make an honest assessment of the time and distance you are going to be putting in and how much food and water you are going to need. Also to be factored in is the level of support for the race. Will there be tables every two miles? Or might the race be unsupported, meaning that you will have to carry everything you are going to need? Not taking the time to learn and size up these aspects of the event can have uncomfortable and even disastrous consequences.

For what I call 'strict running' events like your typical marathon there will generally be tables every few miles as well as strategically placed aid stations. Many races are also held in populated areas, so if something were to happen you at least would not be far from help in most instances.

I get fairly evenly split responses from strict running athletes I speak to, with a fair number carrying nothing and only using support tables. Many brands advertise by stocking these tables so in addition to water, don't be surprised to find bars, goos, and other supplements. A fair number of others choose to use the lightweight 'gear belts' that populate running stores and carry their own nutrition. It really boils down to personal preference considering for yourself the trade off of personalized and always available nutrition against the extra weight and possibility for chafing. There are many events in the endurance challenge community that purposely do not offer these sorts of luxuries, and dealing with this austerity is an art unto itself.

Long distance running athlete Caitlin Alexander discusses her approach to long races and her preferences:

> "I make sure the race has a sufficient amount of water stops and I use those. I never carry my own water unless it's an ultra or it's really hot and the race doesn't have adequate water stops. I sweat a lot and get dehydrated fast. For a half I bring one gel. For a marathon I bring two or three and some other form of nutrition. Lots of marathoners like those gear belts with the little bottles but I don't like having any more weight on me than is needed if I'm trying to run a fast time."

If you are supporting yourself during a long endurance race there are a few factors that you need to consider. The first is how you are going to carry the nutrition you want to use. The second is how your body reacts at high stress levels well into a race (you have been training like you fight right???). And lastly you need to consider the kind of nutrition you will need versus what you know your stomach can tolerate. There is no priority or order to that list, it is all equally necessary and independent.

For instance I know personally that I like to sip water frequently during a race which nets out to a somewhat high fluid consumption. Note that this is generally for events longer than 15 miles and usually longer than 26.2. This means that I bring a water bladder. Partially because I got used to them in the military but also because of their ability to be strapped down tight, I don't mind carrying one. I usually only keep it half full anyway so the whole rig is usually less than five pounds. I know this makes me a little heavier but being able to access supplemented water whenever I want is enough of a boost for me to make it worth it.

When choosing a vehicle for your chosen snackies you need to carefully weigh your options. A gear belt is really lightweight but it doesn't carry very much and may not stand up to copious amounts of mud and violent abuse. Also if you are not used to them they can literally and figuratively rub you the wrong way. A hydration carrier is another option that is popular. It is generally a cut down backpack big enough to snugly fit a water bladder and hose with a few pockets, nooks, and crannies to jam some food, goos, or in some larger models even some foul weather gear.

Hydration bladder carriers are generally pretty tough and

reliable (get used to using a water bladder and tube and look for Army Surplus hydro carriers for even tougher construction). An excellent addition to a water bladder is a waist belt, not for support but for preventing the thing from slapping you on the back the whole race which gets old really fast. The biggest option is some kind of full blown pack. Depending on the event this can range from a cut down minimalist rucksack to an external frame pack for long range expeditions.

This is the wild west as far as selection goes and you are just going to have to test stuff out until you find what works for you. There are two general routes though, one is to pack everything as small as possible to go with the smallest and therefore lightest weight bag. The other option is to go with a bigger bag, dealing with the added weight in exchange for a likely more comfortable harness and more space to easily access your gear which can be packaged as OCD as you like.

Many endurance challenges positively require a full pack, and selecting the right one based on your needs is essential. If you have no previous experience with multi day camping or expedition type events I strongly suggest practicing in any way you can as packing (especially for a high speed and high stress race) is a skill not easily learned and some trial and error is inevitable here. Seasoned endurance challenge veteran Hailie Beam recounts an event where her system broke down for unexpected reasons at a recent Spartan Death Race:

> "I brought 40 lbs of prepared food to death race and ended up only packing & eating protein powder. Sad but true. Although I have a vague memory of someone feeding me half a slice of pizza near the end...
>
> I ended up ditching all of my food except for the powder and a little bit of jerky because my pack was about 65 lbs with only 1/4 of the food I wanted to bring. Luckily, I am never hungry during events & literally have to force myself to eat... so the tasty cookies & cream protein powder worked out pretty well. I also took salt tabs every couple of hours and I vaguely remember taking a shot of this awful Tri powder. Obviously I didn't feel prepared, but I'm not sure I would add more food this year as I need to

save as much space & weight as I can.

I only had access to my "base camp" once for about 30 seconds. I stupidly grabbed a plain red pepper... ate a couple bites and that was it, as I was nervous about getting punished. When I was about to quit, a DNF'er randomly appeared forcing me to eat half a slice of pizza in the rain, and that definitely lifted my spirits... so I might pack some more bacon-flavored jerky this year, but that'd probably be about it.

Next year I'll bring a cooler and put the tuna IN my peppers - ready to grab & go... things like that, but I won't count on it as you never know if you'll have access to the camp. Oh yeah, I need to add that I felt like absolute crap for the next ~5 weeks. Extreme fatigue & mental fog, soreness, etc. It was either the 90 hours of sleep dep, the lack of nutrition or both. So, not sure I would recommend a diet of solely powder! (duh)"

Assessing your body's habits and feelings under high stress

and long exertion is one of the most neglected aspects of training. Well planned and packed nutrition goes to hell when all of a sudden everything looks like limburger cheese because your stomach has gone sour. Loss of appetite is a pretty common thing in severe endurance challenges and it can be a mental block that prevents victory. I am not a physician and so will not try to explain how any of this happens but generally appetite goes sour well into a stressful race and it usually only gets worse with time.

Two tactics I have found effective in dealing with this issue are treating food like fuel (just shove it in and tell your whiny brain to 'can it'), and begin eating steadily long before you are hungry because that hunger will probably never come. I have been told by event cadre after a Challenge that "You were always jamming crap into your mouth". By making snacking a habit during any pauses or breaks I have never had a sour stomach, or many energy issues as far as hunger goes.

Erin Hamilton Prindle has a similar tactic which she describes using during a 10 hour, 12-20 mile GORUCK Challenge:

"I'm a Clif bar, shot blok and Gatorade user. I had to force myself to eat a Clif bar during the Challenge because of what some of the other athletes had talked about just not being hungry but in the long run know I needed it. I know there are probably better things out there than Gatorade but it's definitely saved me on more than a few occasions. Gatorade chews are good, too, and less dense than the shot bloks yet seem to have pretty similar effect - I like those for runs over 8 miles."

There is a pretty common bit of survival and racing wisdom out there that says both that "If you are starving, then you are already in trouble." and "If you are dehydrated, then you are missing more than water." The best tactic for countering this issue that I have found is to get yourself on a schedule however simple or complex where you are systematically refueling yourself with food and drink at regular intervals throughout the event from start to finish.

Endurance athlete Ann Eckler describes past instances and her current approach to events, illustrating how she 'dialed in' what works for her:

"For a 50-miler I did back in June 2013 I was

lucky enough to have access to a drop location twice during the event. So on the direction of my husband I packed a ridiculous amount of food. His thought was to base it on calories - each stop I'd need X amount of calories. Well, I just don't work that way. I, like many of you, have a hard time eating during challenges/long events/long runs, despite the fact that I know I need it.

I was prepared with Clif bars out the wazoo, shot bloks, ProBars, bagels, coconut water, and some "real" food too - baked sweet potatoes, farro w/packets of soy sauce at the ready. At the same drop location, there were also volunteers making PBJ's on the whitest white bread ever, bananas, potato chips. So for the 1st dropbox hit, I grabbed a coconut water (I had run out of regular water miles before), some shot blocks, and then I really wanted a PBJ - just sounded good. Had maybe 1/2 PBJ in the end.

I really could've gone for some

candy/chocolate at that point. Maybe PB M&M's or something like that. The 2nd time I hit the dropbox was at mile 38/40ish and I was definitely in need of real food at that point. I tried the farro, but it seemed SO dry that I couldn't choke it down. Then I grabbed a sweet potato and went on my way. It took a bit of effort to get that down as well, but I did. I also consumed a mix of ProBars and Clif Bars along the way from my stash in my CamelBak. I honestly don't remember how many, but I know it wasn't a lot.

In the events that I've done following that one, I've tried to go more on my gut with what might feel good/sound tasty during different points. I did a Goruck later that same month and got myself a bag of M&M's for that very reason. I'd like to try to get on a path of eating real food for an entire challenge/race, but I'm certainly not there yet. Ditching the bars and blocks is where I'd want to be, but for right now if that's what sounds good to me, that's what I'll be using."

Though the traditional race preparation of 'carb loading' has taken a lot of hits in the recent past, there are still a lot of athletes who subscribe to the approach. In other instances athletes take more incremental steps towards becoming 'fat adapted' (getting most of your race energy from fats as opposed to carbohydrates). This process can be a little hard to get used to but can be made easier by easing into it, this is especially important in preventing problems during the event by completely changing your diet overnight. There is also a quickly growing body of strong evidence pointing to fat adaptation as a much healthier lifestyle in general, not just for athletics.

A frequent participant in endurance challenges, Stephen DeToma puts into detail his hybrid (carb loading and fat adapted diet) approach to events that he currently uses:

> "I usually pregame the day before with a huge chicken parm meal. Before the challenge I've been eating two packs of the caffeinated cliff blocks and I carry water and maybe Gatorade. I generally have something in my ruck as back up like another shot block but often I don't even get to it. For the Lights I

pack way more that I need but that's because I like to share. Popping open a freezer bag of 2 lb of bacon and handing a piece to everyone on the team is something someone did for us in at Santa Cruz 867 and I swore I would do it as often as I could."

Unlike extended running events up to marathon length, endurance challenges often have short breaks, non-running physical tasks, and other opportunities to get extremely hungry. Often in these situations appetite returns with a vengeance and it will often not be satisfied by goo's and all those sugary energy bars. More and more endurance challenge athletes are packing 'real food' to satiate their cravings for hearty fats and salt.

One precaution to packing this way lies not in the nutritional aspects of real food (they are almost universally prefered over processed bars and gels) rather, it is in the physical limitations that all those processed racing foods were manufactured to solve in the first place. Real food often does not contain shelf stable fats (meaning that it will get a little messy if not packed properly). Foods with high water content can freeze solid if it is cold enough and if they are not packed strategically to prevent this. These kinds of considerations lead many athletes to traditional techniques for preparing and transporting food that our kind utilized before the advent of processing and refrigeration.

Athlete Dana Lynn Whitmore talks about the real food that she packs regularly and the learning experience she went through the hard way regarding packing it:

> "I Took some Green Olives, homemade bacon jerky, a mix of raw almonds, pepitas and walnuts, half an unripe banana and sweet potatoes coated in bacon fat (then baked) out hiking in Frozen Head at the Catamount Games. I didn't touch the green olives, and my sweet potatoes froze. Bacon Jerky and nuts kept me happy."

Obviously packing food for your event in this kind of vein takes considerably more preparation and thought than running to a local supermarket and throwing half the supplements aisle in your cart. However, a lot of athletes I spoke to couldn't have cared less about the reduced convenience. On the contrary, they enjoyed the experience of learning new ways to prepare food, shop consciously, and learn about personal nutrition. One of the best favors you can do for yourself as an athlete is learn how to handle, prepare, and cook food for yourself.

Heavy duty freezer bags are an endurance athlete's best friend. Be sure that the closure system is quality and can be operated with mud crusted and freezing fingers. Double bag food if it absolutely should not get wet and you plan on submerging during your event. Wax, parchment, and/or 'butcher paper' is very useful for wrapping meat or burritos; obviously crushing is an issue that necessitates strategic placement (remember to consider the probability that you will be on your back/rolling onto your bag at some point).

Food is also no good to you if you cannot get to it. Burying your food in the bottom of your pack is a great way to set you up to 'starve' (the first world version). There is often not a lot of time to grab a bite and more often than not it'll have to be done on the move. During breaks or stops take advantage of your pockets (you do have pockets don't you!?!?) and stuff some food in them for the foreseeable future so you are not wasting time ripping off your pack everytime you are hungry (or worse just forgoing food altogether).

Once you get the hang of your personal needs and tastes

regarding nutrition you can more effectively tailor your load out to what you are expecting to face. If you are participating in a six hour endurance challenge you will not need to bring 3000 calories of food. With a little experimentation you will easily get the hang of it. Endurance challenge junkie Candace Appleton-Kuntz has long been married to a man who became one of the biggest GORUCK cadre leading events which means that it wasn't hard to find an event with Candace in it. In her experience, once you get comfortable with what goes down well it gets easier to pack what you will want during events:

"My packing of food supplies has varied depending on the event... the first 5-6 challenges I only carried two granola bars and two packs of caffeine sport beans and some bottled water. After that Derek turned me on to his fus stuff which I started carrying in a bottle of water and although I think it's too sweet, it saved me during the DC 7/4 challenge and my Austin Heavy and I also started carrying espresso beans after I was introduced to those.

During my first Heavy I ate nothing except some sport beans, but that's mainly because food was taken away and by the time we got it back I was so dehydrated I couldn't eat. The lights are more for fun, so those have had beer and whatever other goodies and snacks there are. For NOGOA, I packed a lot more food, but Ben Anderson brought bacon and I couldn't get enough of it... had I had that to do over again I would have just brought 2lbs bacon and 2 bags of doritos and a couple granola bars. The MRE was nasty and just made be burp it up for the last part of the event.

Now for my challenges, I will bring a couple more snacks because I love snacks, but I really don't eat too much during the event itself outside of sport beans and the espresso beans - I just need lots of caffeine. And to add to the bacon Stephen DeToma brought me dark and milk chocolate bacon for my birthday light and that may be something I would add to a pack here and there as well.

I had peanut butter foldovers that Abi made me for a couple challenges, I made fun of her in DC for them, but I relished them in our Tulsa and Austin Challenges... even if I did almost choke because there was so.much.peanut.butter..."

One book I highly recommend for anyone interested in getting into endurance challenges is Loren Cordain's *The Paleo Diet for Athletes*. Not only does it give comprehensive nutritional advice for all athletes and specifically for events of varying intensities and durations, but it also dispels a number of myths and old wives tales that persistently stick around in the athletic world. On this note, if there is any area of athletic training that I would advise people to read up on through validated and trusted sources and/or seek professional advice is nutrition. It has the highest potential for hokey ritualistic nonsense which makes taking advice from peers wholesale sketchy at best.

For example, one area that Cordain addresses is hyponatremia which is a significant threat to athletes in the endurance challenge world as their events regularly last more than twelve hours. The common belief in the athletic and military world is that you cannot drink enough water or sports drink, the mantra is "Hydrate hydrate hydrate!" Research has shown that this is a potentially disastrous ritual that can easily dilute your blood salinity down to dangerous levels no matter what you are drinking. An athlete simply needs to drink to satisfy their thirst and no more. We evolved a sense of thirst for a very good reason and as we find out more and more these days, the dark age of medicine's belief that they knew better than evolution is regularly and completely proved a fallacy.

Some notes and updates to this section need to be mentioned to improve the discussion. As of 2015 I have spent a year or so working on 'fat adaptation' and participating in events in ketogenic states. There are terms that are easily abused and I will be crucified by fanatics if I pretend to be absolute about my performance. To that end I was not hooked up to telemetry at every event and I was not followed around by professional nutritionists. I did my best and found sufficient benefit to share the process with you.

Fat adaptation as mentioned before is where you 'dismount' your body from the sugar/carbohydrate ferris wheel. It generally takes a week or two of disciplined effort which is why programs like 'Whole 30' and the induction phase of the Atkin's diet are hard but so successful. This gets your body back into metabolizing fatty acids and ketones instead of sugar and battling insulin spikes/crashes. Sugar is the asshole who cuts in line at the ATM though so it is easy to 'fall off the wagon' in terms of performance.

I essentially follow Cordain's method as close as possible. My everyday diet is between ten and fifteen percent carbohydrate or less (sometimes a lot less). I only start to supplement with carbs ten minutes before my event and during. The amount of carbs (I say carbs instead of sugar because people think of table sugar -see earlier-) I intake goes up as intensity of activity in the event goes up. Ten mile run as fast as possible? Lots of carbs. Three day slow hike on the Appalachian Trail? Small amounts of carbs. I make my own supplements so I can control how sweet everything is. I also use glucose syrup or whole dried fruit to keep fructose out.

I have recommended maltodextrin a lot in this book and I still have a five pound tub of it in the pantry to show for it. It works don't get me wrong and it has pluses over the glucose in being complex and slower acting. Problem is the slow acting (complex) can be compensated for by simply using less glucose in the same amount of water. The other issue was brought up in *Feed Zone Portables* (reference section) in that maltodextrin requires massive amount of water to break down and digest in the body. If I am diluting it in a three liter water bladder that is fine, but I no longer use or recommend concentrating it into 'goo' nor do I use or recommend the commercial stuff. Again, if you tolerate it well and drink lots of water you should be fine.

I have found since greatly reducing my carbohydrate intake that I 'don't need as much of the drug to get the same high' so to speak. During a recent forty mile mountain run I used my normal water bladder cocktail of salt, lemon juice, and glucose. Only towards the end of the race (twenty six miles and on) did I stop at the aid stations and eat some par boiled white potatoes and the slight muscle cramping I was having dissipated rapidly. In previous years I would have had much sweeter water and would have been devouring every aid station on the route.

Be Skeptical

Both the GRT community (people who have completed Goruck Challenges) and CrossFit athletes follow and recommend a number of eating habits with health and athletic performance in mind. The Paleo Diet is particularly popular in the CrossFit community and is frequently attempted by its participants. Because the GRT and CrossFit communities closely overlap many times one frequently sees participants of both advocating Paleo dietary habits. Dana's current nutritional discipline primarily stems from her personal research and objectives but indicates that her interests were initially inspired by her CrossFit compatriots:

> "They definitely influenced me to research diet. I would say the CrossFit Community more than GORUCK, helped push me to a more "paleo" lifestyle. Faction (my gym), has a great crossfit fundamentals course that focuses on teaching you not only the movements, but challenges you to change one small thing in your diet at a time. I was very leery and stubborn at first, because I was used

to the endurance community telling me I needed to shove carbs in my face to do well."

The Paleo diet is often challenging as it contains some pretty intensive restrictions on the typical American dietary fare. Thus incremental approaches like Dana indicated are not uncommon for helping clients ease into the lifestyle change. The exercise and dietary changes that Dana implemented where very successful in the end; in the subsequent time she has lost a significant amount of weight, gained an impressive amount of muscular strength and endurance, and successfully completed even more challenging endurance challenges such as her three (yes three) GORUCK Heavy's (https://www.goruck.com/heavy#.U36tNehX-uY).

How you eat during training and how you eat during events does not have to be exactly the same. Your energy needs will be different depending on the type of training and the event at hand. While some pasta with meat sauce might be OK before a 15k, it will spike your blood sugar and cause you to crash during an hour long Yoga session (many would now say you'll have issues in both situations but I am not qualified to comment). That energy goo or sports drink is ok while running a marathon but will only tack on the pounds drinking it in the gym.

While sponsored athletes need to be seen eating bars and gels during events to get their registration fees paid, chances are you won't see them eating that sugary stuff on the stationary bike at their training center. Study after study in modern nutrition (sports or otherwise) is pointing towards a smaller and smaller need for intaking carbohydrates in the diet. The analogy I often like to use is that carbohydrates are gasoline on a fire, it works great and powerfully, but it is short lived and very often unnecessary. Ben Greenfield has a lot of information to weigh in on the subject and his blog does so extensively. The following is a snippet of his commentary on carbohydrate usage in athletic events:

> "Now, there is absolutely no arguing with the fact that high carbohydrate intake before, during and after a workout can certainly improve performance. So sure – there is at least some logic to the standard recommendation that you should consume a diet which provides high carbohydrate availability before and during exercise.
>
> But while carbohydrates can help you have a

better workout, go faster, or go longer, this only applies to acute, in-the-moment performance. Once you take a look (which you're about to do) at the long-term effects of chronic high blood sugar levels, things change drastically."

This agrees with Cordain's research findings pointing to using carb supplements during high intensity and duration events but not in training and practice events. Unfortunately this means that all that cool colorful stuff you have been eating and drinking during workouts has been largely hurting you. On the positive side it also means you can save a small fortune by switching to water and real food during and after workouts and see significant benefits.

What I have told clients in the past and still do today is that if it is quick and easy, and costs money (especially a subscription) it is probably a load of bull crap. Eating home cooked, simple and natural food while getting a good balance of cardiovascular and resistance training is the only good way to get into athletic (not just aesthetic) shape. In the athletic world it is very much about the hard right over the easy wrong, so be careful about being tempted with something that seems too good to be true, because it probably is.

Motivation for Current and Aspiring Endurance Challenge Athletes

All I am discussing here is what I do personally and what athletes told me they do. You'll have to take my word for it but I didn't know or care what athletes diets were when I interviewed them. I simply chose to interview top finishers and highly experienced veterans of this new world and see what they like to put in their faces. Has my fatty meat eating, carb hating approach to athletics colored my perspective? Yes, of course because it works wonders for me and those I know. I don't claim that this is the only way to do things. I want you to be skeptical as a reader and form your opinions from many sources.

Please use the sources cited section at the end of this book to see where I got my crazy ideas from and check them out for yourself. Especially *The Big Fat Surprise* by Nina Teicholz as it is an excellent investigation comparing the many types of diet that have been shoved at the American people over the decades. If nothing else it will show you just how poor the science of diet has been in the modern age and how we are only just now starting to turn things around.

Many of you reading this probably know a few athletes who can suck down a double helping of pasta dinner, drink a six pack of beer, and still race the next day. I am not arguing against that reality; what I am arguing against is the human desire for everything to be fair and simple. Nutrition like genetics, like love, and like politics is in no way shape or form simple or fair so set that idea on fire and bury it in the back yard. You know you live in a spoiled society when people will get irate with you for making a concept complex and multifaceted.

I am very tempted to simply give the advice of 'never consulting a skinny endurance athlete or a massive world champion body builder about nutrition'. At the risk of sounding like the fat turds who wail "Its all genetics there is nothing you can do!" as they cram in their third cupcake of the day; genetics isn't fair and the world does not care that this upsets you. What does this mean? First it means that if you are new here do not interrupt your 'marathon junky' friend during their pizza/beer lunch and ask them for food advice.

The walking nuclear reactors who live for ultra endurance events were born with a blood sugar tolerance that would put many in a coma. These are the friends who tell you to chill out and eat whatever you want as long as you run eighty miles a week like they do. Truth is you could run like that and still gain a

your genes are arranged even slightly different fi

lifestyle is just not in the cards for most of us.

Here I will get very speculative but to me this seems almost messed up enough to be true. Grant that the endurance community is hard to get into. Yes 5K's are popular but multiple marathon runners who still love life are a tiny sub fraction of the population. Runners even today still eat loads of simple sugars and refined carbohydrates as part of mass printed and subscribed to training programs.

New science shows that much of the population is hit hard by this type of food with sugar spikes and crashes followed by lethargy and sunday football watching on the couch. I would argue that a form of natural selection is taking place. The current paradigm is based around high doses of sugary garbage. Therefore the only applicants to the endurance lifestyle that survive fall into one of two categories. Those whose body mechanics can tolerate that much unnecessary sugar. And those who figure out they can compete using a better nutritional approach because they used their own brains and critical thinking skills to figure out what works for them.

do. Truth is you could run like that and still gain a ton of weight if your genes are arranged even slightly different from theirs. That lifestyle is just not in the cards for most of us.

Here I will get very speculative but to me this seems almost messed up enough to be true. Grant that the endurance community is hard to get into. Yes 5K's are popular but multiple marathon runners who still love life are a tiny sub fraction of the population. Runners even today still eat loads of simple sugars and refined carbohydrates as part of mass printed and subscribed to training programs.

New science shows that much of the population is hit hard by this type of food with sugar spikes and crashes followed by lethargy and sunday football watching on the couch. I would argue that a form of natural selection is taking place. The current paradigm is based around high doses of sugary garbage. Therefore the only applicants to the endurance lifestyle that survive fall into one of two categories. Those whose body mechanics can tolerate that much unnecessary sugar. And those who figure out they can compete using a better nutritional approach because they used their own brains and critical thinking skills to figure out what works for them.

I met numerous would be athletes before I was a trainer and before I knew enough to say anything who just constantly had stomach aches, no energy, and as a result hated running or all exercise. They ate what a magazine or their running junky friend told them worked and they paid the price. At the time they just seemed like 'non-hackers' to me, people too weak to take the pain and commitment to train. But what if in many of those cases we are fooling ourselves with self complements? Maybe those people really are hurting more than us because their bodies are different? All I know is the biggest and best success stories I have seen that last are the ones I see in CrossFit gyms with a nutrition plan/education.

At the other end of the spectrum are the huge muscle heads who seem to gain muscle without effort. Also the unfortunates who gain weight (fat) by just looking at cake can be lumped in here too. Taking advice from these individuals will also be 'tainted'. Mr. Universe will likely be eating so much food that you won't be sure where he finds time in the day to do anything else. The person with a weight issue will be so glucose sensitive that they will need to be on an incredibly restrictive low carbohydrate diet in order to see changes. The former may overwhelm you and the latter may slow

tion for Current and Aspiring Endurance Challenge Athletes

I met numerous would be athletes before I was a trainer and before I knew enough to say anything who just constantly had stomach aches, no energy, and as a result hated running or all exercise. They ate what a magazine or their running junky friend told them worked and they paid the price. At the time they just seemed like 'non-hackers' to me, people too weak to take the pain and commitment to train. But what if in many of those cases we are fooling ourselves with self complements? Maybe those people really are hurting more than us because their bodies are different? All I know is the biggest and best success stories I have seen that last are the ones I see in CrossFit gyms with a nutrition plan/education.

At the other end of the spectrum are the huge muscle heads who seem to gain muscle without effort. Also the unfortunates who gain weight (fat) by just looking at cake can be lumped in here too. Taking advice from these individuals will also be 'tainted'. Mr. Universe will likely be eating so much food that you won't be sure where he finds time in the day to do anything else. The person with a weight issue will be so glucose sensitive that they will need to be on an incredibly restrictive low carbohydrate diet in order to see changes. The former may overwhelm you and the latter may slow you down.

So who do you talk to? Well I would say a nutritionist but until the official science catches up they will likely hand you eight to eleven servings of whole grain bread. One of the most bewildering experiences I had recently was being sternly instructed by a nutritionist easily thirteen points higher on the BMI than me to cut back on saturated fat intake and eat more whole grains. Talk to the middle ground athlete who can run but also has the kind of muscle mass/BFP you are looking for. This person is likely doing the work, tracking nutrition carefully, and earning gains the hard way. Athletic culture like popular culture deifies the .5% and tries to emulate it. Unfortunately this not only cannot happen for most it will infact be detrimental to their training.

Because arguments from personal experience carry little weight formally (despite being stupidly powerful socially), I will try to lay out why I have drifted towards the Paleo lifestyle. By this I mean the reasons apart from that it has worked very well for me. For me a version of independent verification was what initially drew me away from an almost vegetarian lifestyle. While it may not pass in a laboratory setting it is far and away better than the circular, self-justifying garbage reasoning that dominates nutrition (Teicholz).

I am a big fan of the author Mary Roach; her 'dartboard' approach to picking a topic and then investigating every inch of it is fascinating to read about. Even better, from the standpoint of a reader looking for the truth, she is dispassionate and objective in her observations. By contrast most nutritional and dietary investigations/studies of the past decades have been funded or completely controlled by parties with interests riding on the results coming out a certain way. So it was in her book "*Gulp: Adventures in the alimentary canal*" that I started to question the pop science that had influenced my current eating habits.

In the third chapter of *Gulp* Mary bounces between looking at the process of designing and marketing pet food and culturally influenced eating habits. Whether she realized it or not (I suspect not, as she strikes me as someone completely wrapped up in the content rather than the purpose) her coupling of the two disparate subjects paints a very interesting picture for the modern American eater. One thing that jumps out is just how much culture and social bandwagon pressures influence what we think is healthy even when it is in stark contrast to plain as day evolutionary science.

This course of logic is not a hard sell in the endurance challenge community. Probably because by definition you are speaking with people who reject the easy default course and naturally question popular predispositions. I will admit however that a hybrid version of this mentality (monkey see, monkey do) influenced me to overhaul my diet; namely that the fittest and sanest hardcore athletes I met were using a version of a Paleo lifestyle.

By sanest I am addressing the usually out of shape people who will hold up their smart phone with pictures of massive Vegan bodybuilders as some sort of refuting argument. I do not deny that it can work (vegan bodybuilding) I just can't help but point out that it obviously didn't work for the person behind the phone. If you have the drive, focus, and discipline to turn your home into a semi greenhouse with constant rotations of soaking chick peas and fermenting otherwise indigestible lawn trimmings more power to you and I commend your philosophical (if not physiological) choices. I however embrace the ability to sear up pasture raised steak and free range eggs from the local farm with spinach and eat in under forty minutes before rolling out for the gym will a body full of high octane premium energy (fat) and muscle building protein.

In her investigation of pet foods the issue of sweetness comes up. Sweetness has varying implications for different species based on their evolution. Dogs and cats especially do not have much if any taste for sweetness, with a natural feline diet consisting entirely of meat they never developed a love for carbohydrates. One of the reasons we fat humans have fat dogs living with us is we went to great lengths during tin rationing in WW2 to create dry dog food which to this day is largely grains and soy (extremely fattening for both of us). We trick them by coating the food with powdered flavorings similar to the ones we use to trick ourselves into eating trash like cheese curls which otherwise just taste like shame.

Humans and rats share a debilitating 'crack addiction' like affinity for sweetness. And unfortunately simple carbohydrates do the same thing to both of us, namely turn us into fat diabetic blimps. The parallels between disguising pet food and human food to make them cheaper and easier to package, store, and ship was too eerily gross to not cause some serious self examination. I started noticing the arm long ingredients lists on vegetarian items and the acrobatics they had to go through to make the constituents palatable. I think a large portion of todays dietary outlook is a toxic hold over from the

Victorian obsession with order and cleanliness (stitching 'dropped organs' and intense fear of poop). And also the Protestant affinity for the hard road and pain being a virtue/sign of doing it right.

Even more strikingly thought provoking was her stay with the Inuit. She covers it in chapter 3 of *Gulp* as a look into cultural influences on what we find palatable. Again, unintentionally she uncovers major support for flipping the tables on pop nutrition and also the possible problems with pop Paleo adherents as well. Vegetables are a scarce commodity in the harsher parts of Alaska and so is grain. From the outset in thinking like a pop nutritionist these people should be the least healthy and disease ridden people on earth. Rather there are growing campaigns there to drive imported grains and sugars back out because it is killing people at breath taking pace. Keep in mind the traditional Inuit diet is almost entirely meat and much of that being fatty organ meats, eyes, and brain.

There is a reason why predators eat the fatty organ meats and digestive tract of a kill first. It is the most nutritious and calorie dense part of the kill so if they have to bug out they at least got the good stuff. Much of the fringe arguments against meat and used to prop up the food pyramid are based on the lackluster profile of lean muscle meats and a completely fabricated fear of saturated fats. The interesting part is that this cultural fear of organ/variety meats has bled into both camps.

We all know vegetarians argue against meat. Going into detail on that is a whole chapter in another book but suffice it to say their philosophical arguments are sound but there physiological ones are spurious at best. But interestingly I have seen a number of newer Paleo style diets that have not 'made the full connection' so to speak and advocate meat while limiting it to the leanest cuts because they retain the fictional fear of fats. This is a great way to cause a nitrogen imbalance and tempt you to flee back to simple carbs. The reality is that you should look skeptically upon a 'Paleo Buddy' tucking into a filet mignon instead of liver & onions swimming in butter.

I am getting a bit off topic. The point was that Roach had no motivation to sell me fairy tales. Her objective look at the old Inuit culture (mirroring some fit African tribes who eat only meat, blood, and milk) and how modern changes are hurting them made me critically examine my own habits. Before when I mentioned 'independant verification' I meant that authors from varied fields and vastly different interests found the same facts and circumstances concerning a Paleo type lifestyle. This was a major push in that direction for me as nowhere in any of my research did any unbiased party find miracles in ultra low fat, high grain diets like our current American paradigm.

So what if any is the lesson learned? Like the title of this chapter suggests: be skeptical. Never trust a single source as the holder of absolute truth. Explore many different peripheral sources and see what keeps turning up. In the nutrition world if it sounds easy, convenient, and perfect for everyone, then it is almost certainly garbage. The correct answer is almost always going to be a framework based on some basic principles with some custom tailoring to your physiology and plenty of grey area. As I have mentioned before, for the amount of time you spend eating in your life and the importance of it on your performance ignoring or choosing ignorance about food and nutrition is foolish and counterproductive as an athlete.

Motivation for Current and Aspiring Endurance Challenge Athletes

Eating for, and During the Big Event

One of the biggest objections to the Paleo Diet comes from traditional competitive endurance athletes who argue correctly that it cuts a massive amount of carbohydrates from the diet. While not so bad as to hinder athletes in their daily activities (besides the occasional intense craving in the first few weeks), the minimal amounts of easily digestible carbohydrate taken in by eating vegetables and fruit Paleo diet are well below the recommended levels. Especially for athletes preparing for or competing in longer events like GRC's, Spartan Beast's, Tough Mudder's, and races longer than 10K. As one might reasonably expect, athletes on the Paleo diet alter their intake for just such occasions; Dana explains her approach:

> "I use a cycling approach. Most of my training is done paleo. If I feel like I need some extra energy for a long ruck, or workout (or I'm just dragging that day), I'll add quinoa or sweet potato pre-workout. During long events like GORUCK I do add more simple carbs, such as bread, to my pre-event meal, but I try

to balance it out with enough protein and fats to keep me going. I've gotten to the point that I can get by on a couple strips of beef jerky and almond butter packets during a 12 hour event. For the longer events I take pro bars, jerky, mango, and even throw in some gummy bears...because who doesn't feel better when they eat gummy bears?"

An attentive or knowledgeable reader might pick up on the fact that Dana's food choices are based on her objectives or the objectives of the event at hand. While the Goruck Challenge (8-13 hours long) is too long for a carbohydrate starved individual to perform at their peak performance the entire time, that is not the objective. The event is team based and is graded on survival as opposed to what place you come in so experienced veterans will often experiment with just how much comfort they can go without. If Dana were preparing for a 25K with the intention of coming in first place you could be sure that she would be following a structured plan for maximizing her energy stores pre-race as well as a plan to refuel herself during the event.

There are a lot of opinions out there about optimal pre-event fueling and endurance conditioning nutrition in general. One thing is for sure though, showing up for an event calorie deprived and dehydrated is never a good idea. Your approach will be unique to you and is something you'll have to develop to fit your physiology and aspirations. One of the other general constants is that you can stop worrying about your figure during your big event. You will be burning so many calories that short of mashing pure cane sugar into your face as you run you will unlikely to gain any weight when the final numbers are in. As stated before, fussing about your diet during a race can even put your health in jeopardy and hinder your recovery.

As I mentioned before, you need to find out what works for you. Don't buy a bunch of stuff you've never eaten before just prior to your event as you'll just be asking for serious stomach problems. Ultra endurance athlete Jason Spare talks about his nutritional and physiological concerns that he focuses on prior to his events:

> "Go to, would be nutrition and hydration. Days preceding, I load up on fluids and calories to feed "my bank". It's way too late the day of. Electrolyte tabs, pop tarts and now, chia seeds are essential to bring along. A single pop tart has 210 cals, along with

loads of carbs. Slower burning fats and proteins will benefit me much more than gels and power bars (I learned that the hard way by bonking during Ultra. Gear: This has been a trial by fire for me this year. As of now, I won't leave without extra socks and foot care gear. I know with good gear, my pants will eventually dry. Feet: There's something that really boosts the moral, when I have dry, soothed feet. Also, a merino hat does wonders to retain heat, even if I'm wearing wet clothes."

Much of today's leading research in sports nutrition points to listening to natural bodily needs when it comes to hydration. "Drink when you are thirsty and stop when you no longer are." (Cordain) is the KISS method communicated for listening to your body's natural way of signalling the need for water. This flies in the face of numerous classical exercise and training guides that layout complex tables and calculations for determining exacting amounts of fluid intake down to the minute. This newer outlook of drinking when thirsty stems not only from extensive research on real world athletes in competition but also from the growing realization that hyponatremia (the opposite of dehydration) is just as much if not more of a hazard during controlled competitions as dehydration.

Another realization that science has given us that runs contrary to previous thinking is the carbohydrate loading myth. The old paradigm of eating massive amounts of carbohydrates the week leading up to and especially the night before the chosen event has been shown to be at least useless and at most harmful. With the human body's limited storage capacity for glycogen and people's genetic insulin sensitivity varying widely between athletes. Carbohydrate loading oversteps the body's needs and can easily put more susceptible athletes out of the event.

While the process and reality is necessarily complex, in simple terms the body can only store so much glycogen in it's muscles pre-event. The amount of carbohydrate (one fuel source the body uses to create glycogen) that the old paradigm suggested intaking prior to events was vastly too high. It served only to spike insulin levels, store body fat, and give athletes upset stomachs. When asked to explain this simply I find an analogy to filling up your car with gas works well. When you fill up at the pump your car only holds so much to use later. Any extra intake is wasted and causes a lot of problems as it sprays all over your car, the pump, and yourself.

Carbohydrate supplementation is still nearly essential for most athletes in their events though. But what we are finding is that intake just prior to events (ten min) and during is far more crucial and effective than carb loading the night before. Somewhere along the line an athlete looked at a camel and thought "That is a great idea" and the mythical idea and later ritualistic practice of 'carb loading' was born. Unfortunately the human body does not work that way. Our 'gas tanks' with regards to glycogen stores are only so big. All but the most cutting edge completely fat adapted athletes will fail to be able to go without supplementation (and note that they are burning fat, not carbohydrate). Events and physical requirements during longer challenges are at intensities far higher than what our bodies are evolved to handle for prolonged periods of time.

If carb loading worked, trained athletes could pound plates of spaghetti and tackle a 2000m sprint because their phosphagen and glycogen stores would be nearly endless. The reality is that sprints are short because even the most genetically gifted athletes can't store the amounts of the right fuel to sustain such activity for prolonged periods. As it is we are evolved to burn body fat during moderate intensity, long endurance movements with the occasional burst of activity (stalking prey until it tires from running and then killing it). Athletics has made sport of those short bursts of intense activity and much of the science of prolonging it revolves around the optimum intake of fast burning fuels (carbohydrates) to keep those tiny stores of glycogen and phosphagen topped off.

What does this mean for you as an endurance challenge athlete? It means you need to critically analyze the event you are about to train for and take on and strategize your optimal nutritional profile before and during the event. One of the biggest habits to get athletes out of initially is the media reinforced belief that sports products are required for training. The reality is that for many endurance events you want to be as lean as possible as every extra pound of body weight that isn't actively helping you conquer obstacles and cover miles is just dead weight. And one thing that training with sports drinks, gels, and energy bars will do for you is pack on the pounds.

A not totally complete but generally good maxim to follow is that if your workout whatever it may be is less than 90 minutes of moderate to intense exercise in duration then you need nothing more than water to get you through it. For workouts centering on heavy lifts and high muscle fatigue, a high protein/fat, low carbohydrate recovery drink within 30 minutes of the end of the workout is very beneficial if you are hungry. Metabolic testing is done on fasted athletes so the training myth that eating a bunch of protein post workout is a miracle is only true if you are starving. If you workout within a few hours of a big, nutritious meal then you can skip the brotein supplements.

As your workout exceeds 90 minutes you can supplement carbohydrates as needed but be sure to do it throughout the workout and not at the 90 minute mark. After such a workout a higher carbohydrate and high protein/fat recovery drink is a better choice, I like to use frozen fruit, whey protein, and half/half cut with coconut milk for many of mine. The 'drink' aspect is important as your body metabolizes liquid calories more easily (thats why people get fat off of sugary milkshake coffee drinks so fast) and after such intense physical activity your muscles need refueling fast to prevent your body from stealing nutrients from itself.

What is with the fat? Again, a fat adapted athlete largely fuels off of fatty acids. Too much sugar blocks this natural fueling and the insulin released directs the fat to be stored instead of burned. So for my drinks I only add enough carbs in the form of low glycemic berries to restore glycogen. I also add dairy cream (dairy has no negative effects on me so put down your pitchforks paleo freaks, you are allowed to add back in things you tolerate well!) to help metabolize the protein. High protein intake causes nitrogen levels in the body to climb and high levels are toxic.

Fat negates this and levels the body out. Saturated animal fats have no negative effect on cholesterol and don't cause hormone malfunction like unsaturated vegetable oils do. In fact if I know I am not working out again that day and will be taking a rest day I will skip the berries and just stick to protein and animal fat. If dairy messes you up then go with coconut or MCT oil which both work and are delicious.

There are a lot of factors you need to consider when supplementing carbohydrates during your event but whether you need them or not is not one of them. Method of delivery and weight/cumbersomeness are likely the most important aspects to consider and in this case less is quite often more. An important thing to consider is that as the intensity of your activity increases your ability to metabolize solid food reduces. You will need to consider this when packing, and also the tendency for you to prefer to pack less/lighter when activity is intense and prolonged. So the correlation looks like this: The higher the intensity of the event the less solid calories you'll want to pack and the less weight you'll want to carry.

For further information on this subject I highly recommend *The Paleo Diet for Athletes* by Loren Cordain. The other factor that is somewhat less important is length of event. I say 'less' important simply because it is 'added' on to what you should already be doing. As in if your event is intense and long (longer than 12 hours say) you will augment what you would already be doing if the event were say only 6 hours in length. I also classify it as less important because high intensity events that are very long (100 mile trail races for example) allow things like support crews and otherwise facilitate resupply and nutrition whereas mid range intense events are more likely to be unsupported and require you to lug your own nutrition.

As mentioned before, for long and intense events continuous supplementation is key. Eating at intervals is not only inconvenient but ineffective and undisciplined athletes also listen to their reduced feelings of hunger and often forgo eating to their detriment and frequent DNF. A more effective approach is to get your calories in a continuous and easy manner such as mixed into your water bladder. Your average 100oz water bladder can be carried in increasingly lightweight and comfortable racing packs and I find them more comfortable and convenient than bottles. I can easily access my water bladder at any time and its relatively large capacity allows me to refill less frequently.

100oz of water also allows a lot of calories of complex carbohydrate to be mixed in. I prefer using pure maltodextrin because it is cheap, effective, and tasteless/colorless which is more for my hydration bladder than for my taste buds. Mix sports drink concentrate into your hydration bladder for a multi day event and see what happens, hint: it is a sticky, smelly nightmare. This method is also multipurpose as my hydration and calorie supplementation are now facilitated by the same action. A plastic bag with extra powder is light enough and compact enough to shove in next to the bladder if the harness has no storage (but they usually do). Also the powder effectively takes up no space with respect to other necessary gear.

A 100oz water bladder can hold up to four servings of your average pure maltodextrin powder. Four servings is about 268 grams of complex carbohydrate which ends up as a little over 1000 calories. That caloric density and ease of delivery and metabolic acceptance for the total weight (not much more than the water itself) is hard to beat. At high intensities it cannot be bested by solid foods (which won't be processed nearly as well or as quickly to boot).

During longer events you are going to want proteins and fats and this is where some solid food options come into play. But lugging around whole food does not need to take top priority in your kit anymore and every ounce less counts big in many endurance challenges.

Another supplement I have found very effective for longer events and especially for ones with minimum weight requirements is 'Rocket Fuel' (I didn't invent it, that would be stupid). Rocket Fuel is unsweetened applesauce with a few scoops of whey protein mixed in. I usually use a 32oz wide mouth Nalgene bottle filled with the applesauce plus two scoops of whey protein (Vanilla usually). Nalgene bottles are lightweight enough and very durable/watertight and in the widemouth configuration they are easy enough to clean that I generally don't have to worry about them. I suggest mixing the two ingredients together in a bowl beforehand as the applesauce is too viscous to 'shake up' with the protein powder in the bottle itself. You may also find that the mixture is a little thick for your tastes in which case add water until it fits your needs.

For some faster and shorter events you don't want to pack a three course dinner but you also do not want to risk burning out and losing speed. Depending on your approach so far remember the more fat adapted you are before the event the less likely you are to 'hit the wall' or become incredibly hungry during the event. The faster you are moving though, the less fat adaptation matters as it is a lifestyle geared towards going long. For the times when you will be pouring on the afterburners you will want some quick and easy fuel options.

If you do not have the capacity to carry a bottle full of the above 'rocket fuel' recipe and you do not want to carry a bladder full of powder there are other options. I particularly like dates, they are packed full of complex and simple carbohydrates and they store/travel well. Another option I go to now is baking white chocolate. I originally experimented with dark chocolate due to its balance of fat to sugar but the load of tannins and flavonoids delivered with it are a bit much during intense activity. White baking chocolate on the other hand is essentially just fat and sugar and therefore much easier on the stomach. It's weight to calorie ratio is so high that it would be ideal for long term mountaineering trips or wilderness backpacking where ounces count.

One thing to keep in mind when packing for nutritional considerations is that endurance challenge events are often 'unnatural' as far as your body is concerned. Part of the allure and prestige of finishing these events is that you are constantly pushing against your body's desires to slow down or do something else. So why athletes so often push themselves physically against their instinct's desire to take it easy and yet yield to the reduced feelings of hunger that come with intense activity is mysterious. I encounter numerous athletes quitting or just barely finishing events who went ten or more hours with no calories because they 'didn't feel hungry'.

Well as an endurance challenge athlete, one of the first lessons you need to learn for yourself is that many of your feelings are stupid and will get you in trouble. You can overcome some of this lack of hunger by the means previously mentioned by getting your calories through your water source in a mostly tasteless delivery method. But even with this approach sometimes you just have to harden up and make yourself intake calories even if you don't 'feel like it'. Your body is a machine and it needs fuel to run and your feelings on the matter do not play any part in it other than to sabotage your success.

Every athlete over time, experience, and experimentation figures out nutritional strategies that fit their style of event and personal physical attributes. The above mentioned are only what I have found to work well for me and why. I encourage you to take from my experience what you like and add or subtract what works

for you and remind yourself that someone else's approach is no

guarantee of your success. You have to find what works for you.

Don't Sweat the Small Stuff

Planning and time management are often overlooked and neglected factors when preparing for an event. Most of the focus and attention goes to physical training and getting dietary measures zeroed in so that everything feels good for game day. This means that there are a plethora of stories out there involving a highly motivated and steady stomached athlete being late to, or missing their event altogether. All because of some overlooked logistical measure that was not factored into the overall equation.

It is important to factor in your travel when signing up for tough events as. Depending on your planning the travel could have a significant impact on your performance. In general the cheaper you try to go on travel the more stressful it will be. So if you plan on driving nine hours to an event and competing the same day just realize that you are at a significant disadvantage. The person who sprung for the plane tickets and flew two hours (of which 1.5 was nap time), all other things being equal, will have the edge. This can have at the very least an impact on your disposition and irritability during your event, which for some venues can be a detriment.

Travel can add some significant logistical and physical constraints to your event planning. Foreseen or not, travel taxes the body and car travel continues to be one of the leading causes of injury and death to people. Stack on top of that reality the fact that you have just competed in a grueling endurance challenge that has deprived you of calories, water, sleep, and possibly self esteem and you have a deadly cocktail that driving nightmares are made of.

The reality is that flying is expensive and so the frugal amongst us will attempt to drive when we can. There is no question that driving is more dangerous, but it can often be much cheaper. If you are a budding champion on a budget then there are some planning steps that I consider mandatory for success when road tripping to events. On the other hand, if you are just a little cheap and your event is more than sevenish hours drive I would highly recommend flying.

When committing to car travel make sure to plan in rest on the way to the event as well as back from it. I made the rookie mistake of cramming six and a half extra hours onto my first attempt at GORUCK's 48+ hour Selection event by driving straight down to

Jacksonville Beach without any pre-event nap time in the schedule (big mistake). It greatly contributed to my failure to complete the event. After your event, make sure to rest for at least a few hours before driving home. You may be hopped up adrenaline but you are likely far more exhausted than you think you are.

Help yourself out by not scheduling any 'do or die' plans for right after the event back at home. The event is over and you should not be rushing home, take your time and take breaks. You can also do yourself a favor by carpooling. Get some like minded buddies together and share the driving responsibility and gas money. This is a safer and more cost effective way to travel by car (plus you can use the HOV lane!). Also remember to do the math, if you are not a roughneck road tripper and refuse to go without hotel rooms and sit down restaurants on your trip then you may find yourself paying just as much if not more than a plane ticket to get to your event.

GORUCK events tend to force participants to keep it simple. You know what city you'll be in but not any specific location until about four days out. This keeps things interesting and prevents people from making intricate and impractical travel/party plans. In defiance of this Tim Rosenberg managed to get his plans tangled

Motivation for Current and Aspiring Endurance Challenge Athletes

up leading up to his GRC in Boston. Despite this gum up in planning Tim managed to make things work and was able to keep from letting the scheduling nightmare affect his attitude towards his classmates during the challenge.

Tim:

March 16, 2013 0100 – whenever

Boston St. Patrick's Day. GORUCK. My first Challenge in a major metro. This only marks the third Challenge that I've completed….and by far it was the biggest. So here goes nothing. Photos are courtesy of Andrea Towle our dedicated Photog who was with us the entire time.

Arrivals and Welcome Party

This was supposed to be easy. Take the Friday train to Boston, do a Challenge Saturday morning, sleep and come home on Sunday. Work called the week before; I'm needed at the Virginia office for a bunch of Really-Important-Meetings with Really-Important-People. Ok…I can be flexible (those that know me know this is a blatant lie. I'm a terribly anxious traveler). I'm traveling with 32 pounds of bricks, duct tape and a 25+ pound, 42 inch war hammer. I have my train tickets already booked...so how can I get from Dulles to Boston on Friday and return to Lancaster on Sunday by 4:30 pm for a multi-family dinner?.... this is what I came up with...

1. One of my work mates still works in Chantilly. He will drive up to PA on Wednesday before the Challenge.

2. Thursday he will drive me and my kit down to Chantilly.

3. I'll attend the meetings Friday, take the 4:55PM flight to Boston, cab it down town.

4. Do Challenge

5. Take train home to Lancaster and hitch or walk home from the train station.

   I'm sure I couldn't possibly put any more moving

parts to this if I tried. Thursday comes, I've business suit, Challenge equipment and bricks all ready to go. At 5pm, I find out most of the Really-Important-People can't make the meeting. I grab my team, go out to dinner and stall until 7pm; waiting for the remaining to drop out or confirm. No word. I bail. Stay in Lancaster and go back to the original plan of train up and back from PA.

Friday

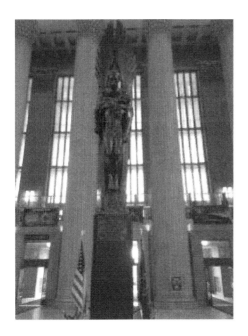

Philadelphia's 30th Street station.

Nice and easy. Gear up, drive to Amtrak station and head north. It was a really relaxing ride. I talked to some very nice people on the way up. As I approached South Station in Boston, the nerves began to kick in again. I go into auto pilot; and head to the hotel and drop gear. With that done; I head to the start point in the daylight and get my bearings. Done. Find a CVS and load up on water. Done. Find dinner. Eat.

No luck attending the 'Before' party. I rack out in the hotel room; wake up, kit up and head to the start point...and there's a ton of people. 102 to be exact, plus Cadre, Shadowers and Photographers. I run into a couple from Facebook; hand Gretel (a 30lb hammer) around and generally hang out....then the fun begins. The first couple of hours are again a blur.

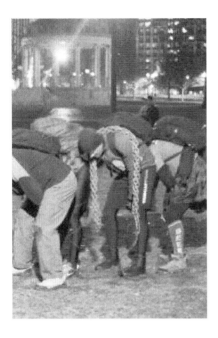

Welcome party.

We do some general warm ups and then divide into Alpha, Bravo and Charlie groups. I'm in Charlie (along with 40 other people) and we get Cadre Garet. We move off to our own corner of Boston Commons and start the welcome party. Pushups, squats, flutter kicks, sprints, buddy carries and more. The fun begins. I'm weak again with the buddy carries; I can get my partner to one end of the field, but have to piggy back him on the return. After an untold number of minutes (hours?) we form up and move out.

strangers, a massive green chain, Gretel, and our Flags.

The Tour

And so begins the tour of Boston. Chinatown, State House (broke formation here to go explore), Quincy Market and Faneuil Hall. City Hall steps (sideways crab walks up and bear crawls down), Old North Church, Bunker Hill Monument (morning calisthenics with Deadmau5). Long haul to Fenway, Emerald Necklace for a log pickup and dip in the water. Boston Public Library (warm bathroom). Boston Harbor. Route back to Boston Commons and take casualties (only the big people die of course). And then we are done.

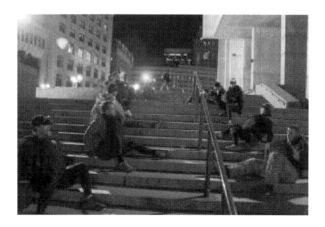

Crabwalk up the City Hall steps

Boston. The birthplace of Freedom. I'd read about some of the places. Faneuil Hall where speeches of freedom were heard, Old North Church where Paul Revere started his famous ride, Bunker Hill (actually Breed's hill) where few stood before many and changed the world forever. It was humbling to stand where a handful of militia took a stand against the mighty and powerful British Empire. For this amazing tour of Freedom, I thank Cadre Garet.

The Team

A team of 41 is very different than the group of 9 from Columbus. We started with two weights (the chain and Gretel). We pick up sandbags and half a railroad tie. We shift weights, change Team Leaders and kept moving. Missed time hacks are rewarded with PT; almost always push ups. We do our pushups to the cadence of 'Attention to detail'/'Teamwork is key' and 'One Team, One Fight'. In the beginning it was just words. Over the night and the miles names are exchanged and stories are told. Packs are shifted when people needed a break; we rotate through the team weights.

At the crab walk we had our first drop. The group broke into two columns, faced each other and began crab walking up the stairs sideways. I was near the end of the one column when one of the women stepped out. She was done; 'I can't do this' was uttered. The group closest to her rallied. Her pack was passed up the column, encouraging words were shouted and she did it. As the group continued on, 'One Team, One Fight.' became a reality. The miles and hours pass, a couple more try to quit (we don't let them). Packs are rotated some more; the strong carry more, the steady lend a hand and the light of heart keep the smiles going.

Motivation for Current and Aspiring Endurance Challenge Athletes

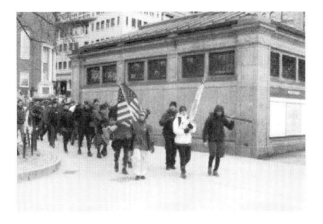

Almost there.

41 people started. 41 people finished.

The End

At the end we pose for our pictures and receive our patches. As Cadre Garet hands me my patch, I hand him the Dirty Dozen patch I wore for the Challenge. I explain that I completed this to honor Sgt. Park. Turns out Cadre Garet knows his brother. I share a few drinks and head back to the hotel. Thank you to Cadre Garet, Sgt. Park and the men and women of #453.

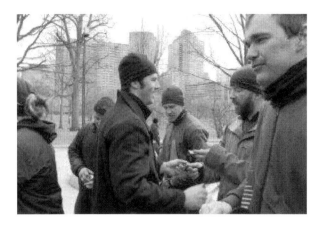

As with training, it is best to keep things simple when planning the background logistics for your event. You'll want to plan in the least number of variables and 'moving parts as possible so that there is less chance of something not working out. Such issues can adversely affect your ability to make your event in the first place or your performance when you do make the start line. Again a great approach is to research whatever resources the event makes available to the public. They have likely answered a lot of questions and dealt with a lot of participant issues and subsequently put up a FAQ page for your convenience. Likewise, talking with someone who has completed the event previously will likely reveal nuts and bolts of the logistical side of the event you can't easily research (like parking).

Friends and Battle Buddies

Buddies make the world go round and a good partner (or group) can make the difference between a steely faced, no fun suck fest and an enjoyable event full of belly laughs and encouragement. Depending on your competitive style (and if you are even trying to be competitive at all) it can make all the difference to have a familiar face to suffer through the event with. Not only will you have someone to talk to during the event but you will also be able to carpool to the event to boot. Christian Nelson describes how having a buddy with him made a difference during his experience at World's Toughest Mudder:

> "I realize this wasn't part of your question, but it's also a huge help to have a 'buddy' at WTM. I ended up running the entire event with Justin Willett, famous in TM circles for his Hello Kitty backpack. Where I may have been weak, he was strong and vice versa. We pushed each other to continue, and to do more than we might have if we were solo. You aren't allowed a 'crew' so being next to each other in the pits and helping each other out was huge for us."

Stories like this are especially prevalent for 'experience' goal setters rather than competitive goal setters. People who set a goal to 'show up for and finish' an event are likely to get more fun and motivation out of bringing along a buddy than someone who is looking to take first place or beat a specified time standard. For most new events I prefer to bring some friends and 'just finish' the event and then decide afterwards whether or not I want to come back and try to tackle the event competitively. Sometimes this approach is not an option but there is often a lot more wiggle room in these sorts of events once you've paid your registration fees.

There are not many things that bring a team together as effectively as shared misery. When you are in a group of individuals all going through the same deprivation and hardship your evolved altruisms kick in as your brain screams at you that working together and cooperating tends to make things easier. Even when you are not supposed to help out fellow participants the want to do so is still there and can be very strong. Such is why stories of subtle and even secret acts of camaraderie in completely individualistic conditions are so commonplace in the endurance challenge community.

Part of the initial screener class for GORUCK Selection (an event where candidates are not allowed to interact or speak to one another) endurance athlete Spencer Guinn talks about the bond between candidates that was formed regardless of the event requirements:

"It's difficult for me to explain how well our team "meshed" together under the crucible provided by the Cadre. Even though by the end we were sleep deprived, hungry, hallucinating, injured, etc we were all focused on finishing together. All remaining water was shared. All remaining food was shared. There was no longer individual equipment. If one of the team needed something, it was immediately offered. No arguing, and decisions were discussed and made. Yes this was an "individual event," but it was obvious that we were in it for the team. I have the utmost in deep respect for every member."

This sort of organic teamwork and camaraderie creates an interesting dynamic in events with specific rules and procedures. You want to help your teammates out as best you can but have to be able to let go if they drop out. If you become too attached to someone and forget about your original goal then their dropping out can have a seriously negative effect on your ability to push on towards the finish line.

It isn't necessary for your friends to do the event with you to receive benefit from them being there. Many events abide spectators and many others are happy to employ volunteers for help at aid stations. The availability for this sort of support goes back to cultivating a group of friends ready to support one another. I have a group of local endurance athlete friends and we have an unspoken agreement that we will come out and crew for each other at events whenever possible. Of course we prefer to all participate but sometimes that is just not possible and having the support regardless is a big morale booster.

If your friend scratches your back then you need to put in the effort to scratch theirs back. Never take your crew or aid station volunteers for granted. Their job is unglamorous, difficult, and outside of the focal point of attention. If you have a friend willing to do this sort of service for you then you definitely owe back the same. If they happen to not be into endurance challenges then you need to find another way to pay them back.

Building a social base in the endurance challenge community can net you and your friends some interesting opportunities. Most athletes in this field have diverse interests in outdoor and indoor hobbies alike and may invite friends to partake. As discussed before getting too sucked into endurance challenges can lead to burnout and overuse injuries so it is nice to have some calmer adventure hobbies to turn to from time to time. You won't be able to win endurance challenges forever so make sure you have something interesting to do with good friends when that time comes.

Why Are You Doing This Anyway?

Motivation is a personal thing but a common thread in the world of extreme endurance challenges. Many of the events out there will push the average individual far outside their comfort zone and require vast amounts of physical and psychological reserve in order to hope to do more than merely survive. This is why so many individuals at these events have such great background stories and driving purpose. Often this inspiration and drive spreads to those who are in close contact with these individuals and it is not uncommon to see others alongside these unique people at events because they felt duly inspired to push themselves and help ensure their friend's success.

A fair amount of those who participate in endurance challenges do it for the motivation and inspiration they get and give to those they meet and interact with during the events. For these sorts of people competition is not the focus and where they end up in the stats is entirely separated from the fulfillment they get post event. They set a personal goal and help out those they come across. Events like Tough Mudder and the GORUCK Challenge emphasise and in many cases demand this sort of attitude to the exclusion of competitive gains. As he says here, this is one of the reasons Christian Nelson got into GORUCK events as his favorite flavor of endurance challenge:

"For me the allure is because it's non-competitive. I don't get joy out of being better than the guy next to me, just better than I was last time. I mentioned earlier how the people were the reason I enjoyed this stuff so much. I find in the more competitive events (Spartan) that the people aren't as much fun to be around. I think it's different for everyone."

Others go into training towards these endurance challenges as a benchmark or milestone in a lifestyle and fitness shift in their lives. Performing well (or simply making it through) the event becomes a driving force for getting into the gym or adhering to better nutritional choices. This is then often augmented by the social nature of these events.

These motivated people encounter and link up with like minded participants and often make lasting friendships. Many times these connections go well beyond acquaintances and go onto have a significant impact on the lives of all involved. Again Christian talks about how his initial motivation to get back into shape resulted in close friendships that helped stabilize his life during future challenges:

"Three years ago I was fat and lazy. Since I was twelve years old I was always "chubbier", but pushing 280lbs and not fitting into 40" pants I was unhappy. The straw that broke the camel's back was seeing myself in my buddy's wedding album. I decided to take it slow. My initial goal was just to work out three times a week, at least an hour, for three weeks.

In three weeks I'd dropped fifteen pounds and that was all the motivation I needed. I ended up losing seventy pounds in six months. A buddy showed me a Tough Mudder YouTube video and the next day I registered. I had never even run a 5k event before the day I did the Tough Mudder. I instantly fell in love with the experience, the camaraderie, and the people. That year I did three

Tough Mudders and other assorted mud runs.

The thing was my personal life was starting to fall apart. My marriage was on the rocks due to my wife becoming a cop. We did class 131 in Boston over St Paddy's Day weekend and it revived our relationship for a bit. It didn't last, I ended up kicking her out.

I signed up for Hartford and Charlotte GORUCK Challenges. Fast forward, May 30th, my wedding anniversary, Horse posts on my Facebook wall inviting me to be a part of TeamFARM. The people I met during these first few challenges and TeamFARM were there for me during a year where I should have been at my absolute lowest, but because of them I had purpose. It's the people; the friends made. Seeing people push past what they thought they could do."

Because of the intensive training commitment involved in being competitive in such events these background stories of personal trials and tribulations are quite common. Taking this in mind one might look to such endurance events as a venting opportunity in order to redirect focus from particularly bleak areas in life. Though some athletes ooze motivation and enthusiasm on a genetic level, many of us do not. For this reason it is important not to trivialize personal back stories like Nelson's. Sometimes it is an experience in life or a change we desperately want to make that can help us cross that deep divide between those that do and those who do not.

CrossFit coach and Memphis Tennessee native Dana Lynn Whitmore is a female athlete with extensive experience in both conventional and unconventional endurance challenges. She has a plethora of half marathons under her belt along with experience in structured fitness camps. In recent years she has taken her training to the next level and tested herself with intense endurance challenges from Spartan Race and a number of the longer team based crucibles put on by GORUCK.

Past athletic experience is a major indicator for ability/willingness to engage in physical challenge later in life. Many individuals are active in grade/high school and then become sedentary when the stressors of college, marriage, and career hit in succession; fewer still manage to hold a 'steady state' of physical activity throughout their lives by transitioning school sports experience into time at the gym and recreational activities like Golf and charity runs. Fewer still are engaged and fond enough of their activities in their youth to the point that they are motivated to escalate their activity levels for physical, mental, and social gain. Dana provides an excellent case study in this last category as she explains her athletic past:

"I have always been fairly active; I played softball and was on the pom team in Junior High and part of high school. In college I didn't do much - I went through the motions at the gym just to stay thin. Elliptical for an hour, that sort of thing. In 2008 I started running races. Anything from a 5k to a half marathon. I also started a fitness boot camp. I picked up a dumbbell for the first time in my life (to actually exercise with) at that point. The motivation was pretty selfish. I had a beach trip coming up and wanted to look good. I stuck with that boot camp program until I found GORUCK in 2011. A lot of people that were in

GORUCK talked about crossfit, and I wanted to check it out."

After her first GORUCK Challenge class 097 in Memphis Dana was awoken to the fact that moderate to intense cardiovascular training and organized fitness classes would not quite cut it for unconventional and intense events. The average GORUCK Challenge (whatever that means) is between eight and twelve hours long and can cover distances of twenty five miles and beyond. All the while participants haul all manner of objects like trees and rucksacks with forty pounds of bricks in them. When asked if post Challenge she had felt prepared for the endeavor she responded:

"Absolutely not! I was completely unprepared. The only thing I had going for me during that first challenge was endurance and the mental strength not to quit. While I did get under the log for a good amount of time during that challenge, I had no extra strength to carry team weights, coupons etc."

If you still have the itch it is important to remind yourself that you can always go up, meaning that there are more challenges to tackle and more worthwhile causes to take up. Unless the challenge you have been preparing for is to stride onto the Vigrid Plain there will be life after your event and you must prepare your mind to stay busy once it is all over and the trophy is mounted on the wall. Especially if the event is one of the popular endurance events (Spartan Race, Tough Mudder, GORUCK) you will likely make friends that you can reminisce with afterwards and hatch new and crazier plans with. Dana describes the experience:

> "Haha! It's an escape from real life...and you get to be with awesome people that you tend to have a lot in common with. It's hard to go back to everyday life/work after an experience like that. Not to mention most people don't understand what you just accomplished, so you can't really talk to them about it after."

Many of these kinds of events have group pages on the internet that connect veterans and allow people to relate their experiences to each other as well as advise those hoping to take on the next challenge. Foresight is really the tool most needed here. Realize that after training and mentally focusing on a single event for weeks and months of your life you may feel temporary (remember, temporary) feelings of lost purpose and direction. Or set yourself a small number of related goals that will happen in succession so that when one event is done there is always another one on the horizon.

With a huge majority of the American population ceasing nearly all exercise related activities after grade school where PE is generally a required activity. This is also when parents are more likely to encourage extracurricular sports activities if for no reason other than to get kids out of the house. It is little wonder that a common theme among those getting into the endurance challenge lifestyle revolves around them reclaiming past activity levels. If it weren't for the disproportionately small population of the endurance challenge community this might be an encouraging thing. Sadly though these inspired individuals are the tiny minority in the growing population of land whales.

Matt Ogle is one of those few who fought to reclaim the daily strength and endurance expenditure of youth and worked his way back into an active lifestyle. He eventually became a major figure in the GORUCK community by completing numerous events including the inaugural 'Heavy' at Ft. Bragg NC, 25 hours of serious physical hardship that saw an attrition rate of 50%. He discusses his journey back to fitness and his current goals:

"I was very active in high school. Played soccer three seasons a year and did camps in the summer. My sport of choice once I got to college was beer. After college I got into running to keep myself busy and signed up for my first race to impress a girl haha. That didn't work out but I caught the running bug and stuck with it for races and the stress relief of the training.

The current goal is GR Selection. That will be the next thing I do. After that, I'd like to run a 50 miler and a few other big events like Spartan Death Race. But that's after Selection."

To participate and compete with the best athletes that take part in these competitions physical training has to move beyond a program or a isolated train up period. For many serious athletes physical fitness is a devoted hobby for them, that can at times become a driving obsession. While there are innumerable hobbies out there that could be argued to be far worse for body and soul than honing physical fitness, friends and family tend to only tolerate driving obsessions for finite periods of time. For this reason making fitness a continuous hobby bares it's fruits in that it spreads the effort and preparation out over manageable time chunks across your schedule. It also makes you less prone to training injuries as 'fast and steep' train ups are particularly hard on the body.

Science has shown that regular exercise goes a long way towards preventing disease, relieving stress, and improving attitude. This is why taking the long view and getting yourself into a steady state of fitness where you can jump into your event of choice without a massive train up will not only contribute improvements to your everyday life, it will prevent you from annoying those around you with overly intensive obsession like training periods in the weeks leading up to an event. Matt Ogle describes his mindset and outlook on his athletic training:

"It can be a major stress reliever. It's a good diversion when there are other big things going on in my life. But at the moment, with selection training being the big thing going on for me, it can be as much a source of stress as a relief from it.

They're definitely a positive hobby. I could see them becoming an obsession if I found a good training group that introduced some competition into my training, but at the moment, training mostly alone, it's just a hobby. I've always had a pretty deep competitive streak, so in the right situation I could see that resurfacing."

The endurance challenge world is not entirely competitive, many events like Tough Mudder and the GORUCK Challenges do not have top finisher spots or even formats that support such finishings. Regardless, athletes have a tendency to compete with themselves before and during the event. This can be a major motivator to get out and train, but it can also blind the individual a bit with regards to the regular responsibilities of life. So be sure to take care to train hard while keeping your priorities straight.

Unconventional Families

One of the recurring themes I come across when asking people why they love pushing themselves in the world of endurance challenges is the people that they meet. Hard times bring people together and we are lucky enough to live in a society where hard times are not forced upon us daily by life. Rather the majority of us get to volunteer for some adversity that fits into our schedule. While that sounds superficial I would still take a Spartan Beast over a tuberculosis epidemic to build my character any day and am thankful for the option.

These trials of adversity and physical challenge have a way of bringing people together both on and off the course. There are large thriving communities of individuals who identify with others from the same background endurance challenge. These communities quite often go beyond simply reminiscing about past events by raising money for charitable causes and lending a helping hand to community members in need. Best friends and close loved ones alike have been found and maintained through communities like these. These both perpetuate participation in these events and often inspire others to earn the right to join these tight knit communities.

There is a difference between friends and 'digital friends'. Friends on Facebook are not the same as friends you know from personal, face to face interactions. One of the great things about participating in endurance challenges is the fact that you will have little choice but to make interactions, be on teams, and generally have massive amounts of face time with other people.

Some of these fellow participants will have an impact on your life and may even become lifelong friends you regularly keep contact with. These are going to be the people in both your thoughts and reality who are going to motivate you when times are tough. When victory is on the line and your mental faculties are stretched to their limits, the opinions of your 'digital friends' will have little effect on driving you. The motivation imparted by friends and family in person however will be vivid and powerful even in the depths of fatigue and deprivation.

Endurance challenge athlete David Thomas went beyond personal training for GORUCK Selection by making friends and close connections. These relationships not only provided him with advice and techniques from other experienced athletes but also gave him a close network of people who cared about his success and who he did not want to let down:

> "Having others know what you are doing holds you accountable. It's easy to skip training or not push when its only you doing it. But having others (training partners, significant others, whatever) on board with you keeps you on track. Also, I sought help from anyone I could – read all the AAR's, talked to cadre, talked to finishers and non-finishers. I gathered all the information I could and made it work for me. Different things work for different people, but I didn't discount anything."

Just like with any family though, when the gathering is big enough personalities tend to collide. It is simply a social law that as a group gets bigger the overall personality deviates towards chaos. This is when the maturity and level headedness of key group members is tested in their efforts to bring the focus back onto what is most important. In his excellent reflection, Richard Sanders makes an effort to do just that, bring focus back to the core message. In his effort to remind everyone why they are there, Richard gives the reader some great insight into his own take on the meaning of the community as a whole and why people are drawn to support each other when coming from these sorts of shared experiences:

Richard Sanders

At the end of the day, I hope the Challenge taught every one of you a lesson that I feel is important in any team exercise: no matter what your motives were in sign up, (whether it was to test your own limits, something as superficial as earning your Tough patch, or to prove something to somebody) when you're at that Challenge, the Cadre don't care why you are there. As far as they are concerned, your reason for being there is the person to your left and your right. You are all they have and they are all you have. If you don't give up on them, they won't give up on you. And this is the gap; this mentality of camaraderie is the gap that needs to be bridged between servicemembers and civilians. GORUCK is doing an excellent job of trying to do just that through venues such as 'War Stories and Free Beer' and the Challenge itself.

I think back to my first of now seven GORUCK Challenges, class 141 with Cadre Lou and Chris Stokes. I was barely a few months out of the active Army (prior 13F) and was having a miserable time adjusting to civilian life. 21 years old at the time, everybody I had graduated with was still at home, at the bars, doing the same thing. Whilst in the past four years, I had to grow up through trial by fire, had more responsibility than these people would ever comprehend, and as a result felt like I'd never fit in anywhere again. I had about lost hope in society until I met my fellow GRTs and witnessed firsthand that there is, in fact, hope for people like me... people like us. I was 138lbs soaking wet for my first Challenge. To date, it was still my most miserable one, but my team would never let each other down.

At the end of the Challenge, Lou said one thing to us that rings with me to this day: "Treat everything you do as a Challenge. No matter what it is in life- if you treat everything like you did this Challenge, you will excel".

Those words resounded with me on the way home. Had those words not been spoken to me, I may not have the GPA I have, may not have completed the classes I have, may not have maintained the income I have. And had I not done any of that- let alone what I did prior with the military, I would not be here now, happier than I have ever been in my entire life.

GoRuck Tough is a community of go-getters that prove every day, that there is no Challenge too difficult. If you give this community a task, it will accomplish that task- and often over deliver. We leave none of our own behind. Feel free to show me any community besides veterans themselves where, no questions asked, you have a place to stay if it ever came down to it anywhere in the country. 'Normal people' do not have this. By pushing yourselves outside of your comfort zones, you earned more than a Tough patch; you earned entry into a tight knit family.

Family isn't about genetics or blood. Family is about who you care about and who cares about you. My biological family decided to tell me to go fuck myself with my enlistment, and that doesn't sadden me a bit. The fact I can choose my own family, and have chosen my own family, makes me happier than having a blood family will ever make me. I've been on the giving and receiving end (and I know one of you is going to make a joke about that) of the help spectrum here, and to me, that's what family is. Most people in our society with 'blood families' just go through the motions because they feel like they have to.

Whether it was during the Challenge itself or at some other point in your life, all of you have had to fight demons. We've all had that pivotal point in our lives, whether it was during the Challenge or not, that we decided "No, fuck this. I'm going to make shit happen." For me, that was when I was a 16 year old fat loser in high school. I had a ridiculous crush on this really pretty girl named Lauren Fay in high school. She wouldn't have dreamed of giving me the time of day. My 'Challenge' was my enlistment, completely turning my life around. I fell off the face of the earth for four years and saw her again at a half marathon. Those four years were my Challenge, my decision to change things for the better.

Last year on Memorial Day, I came across a few major realizations: I could care less about my birthday and cared entirely about my brothers I served with. I spent time with my family, James Montgomery (whose wife taught Jason McCarthy, and got me into GORUCK in the first place,) and I regret nothing. GRTs would get this, 'normal people' would not.

For all we bitch at each other, never forget one thing. You're all part of a community that does amazing things for each other. While at the age of twenty two, most people I graduated with are preoccupied with their sole sources of charity work being bar crawls (i.e. nothing whatsoever) if we GRT's make fundraising objectives on the Tough page, shit gets done. An old teacher of mine and I ran a fundraiser for Sandy; we got three donations and all were from GRTs. I set up a fundraiser for SWSF for the Challenge this weekend with a goal of raising $500, and it was met within three hours.

We give each other the courage to accomplish tasks, whether they are fundraisers, support for families dealing with loss, cancer, Sandy, anything. To me, that is a million times more of a family to me than a blood family ever would be. There are older GRTs that I view as parental figures that have given me timeless advice (yes, outside of Papa Lou's wisdom from earlier) and there are GRTs I view as the closest friends I've ever had outside of the military.

Were it not for the advice given to me by some of these GRTs, I don't need to name names, because they know who they are, earning my patch would have never happened. My demons would have eaten me alive and I would have VW'd from the entire situation, and given up on the best thing that's ever happened to me. The support I have received from this community throughout numerous events this past year; Sandy, military related circumstance, mentally, academically... has just been more than I can put into words, and I literally have no idea where I'd be without you people.

So at the end of the day, never forget that by completing your Challenge and being on this page, you're part of a family better than most people will ever be able to comprehend. Treat every day like a Challenge and great things will come to you all. We take care of our own and we never leave each other behind.

Team Death Race

Death Race is an event defined by pushing participants way outside of their comfort zones in unconventional ways. Changing schedules, last minute packing list changes, bizarre packing list items, outlandish tasks, and verbal and emotional abuse are just a few of the challenges participants face as they strive for the finish (which is entirely unknown to them). This hardship creates camaraderie amongst the participants and the larger spectating community. This effect creates a drive to support the participants and encourage them in any way possible and has resulted in some excellent stories of inspiration. Multiple time Death Race finisher Mark Webb describes his most recent experiences at the Team Death Race:

Mark Webb

Even getting there was problematic. At first I couldn't make it due to parenting obligations and so my original team disbanded. Fast forward a week and the timing changed my obligation changed and I could make it.

Even better, one of my best friends and partner in crime in so many challenges and at Selection Screener, Francev needed someone. Stars aligned, and I was on my way to Pittsfield.

As usual the race was filled with frustration, irritation and impatience for the first half but more so was filled with jokes, innuendo and laughter. My team was the shortest in cumulative height. We are all 5'6" to 5'7". We were also tenacious and motivated. As we moved towards the race portion our intensity increased and we all drew power from the other team members. There was never an argument, and always support.

The second to last task was a hike from Pittsfield to Killington. We were the first "walking" team there by far - a testament to the thousands of miles we have all accumulated under a weighted ruck. We didn't endure the rain, we embraced it. We wished it would start to suck more. The final task was to complete the Spartan Ultrabeast; a marathon(+) distance obstacle race up and down (repeatedly) one of the steepest mountains in the

North East. We agreed to stay together as a team unless our pace was vastly different. I had shed more pack weight than my team and so forged ahead and spent most of the race alone and yet not alone.

The thing that keeps coming back is how amazingly supportive EVERYONE was. All through the UB (ultra beast) words of encouragement came from regular racers "Go Death Racer!" from those that didn't know me and "Go Webb!" from those that did.

I personally was running behind the caloric curve and often asked strangers for food. They provided without question. I ran past one racer and he was already holding out a bag of sports beans "Take this! Good luck".

Special thanks to Kristy, Adam, David, Todd and Andy who fed me, asked how I was and when I said "fine" got out of my way. Also thanks to Ekaterina, Amelia and Don for unexpected beers mid race. Not good for hydration but huge for motivation. I am sure I missed some folks so I thank you all too. Its hard to put into words how amazing the DR community is, and I was even more amazed at the generosity of complete strangers to a not-perfectly prepared man in need.

Because I ran light I was able to run an extra 6 mile loop (yay :/) which put my team ahead of me at one point. Being able to catch up near the end and cross the finish line as a complete team was the icing on the cake.

The skull is nice but the memories of all the people, and all those moments transcends everything else.

Death Race = Life Race.

Accountability

One thing you come to find when hanging out with habitual marathon runners and classical ultra endurance athletes is that they are necessarily narcissistic, self absorbed people. I know exceptions, but not many; hang out with them for long and you will be lucky to stray the conversation away from their personal preferences for shoe purchases and archaically religious carb loading rituals. If you have ever talked to someone and been pretty sure they were just staring straight through you waiting for their turn to speak then you know what I am talking about.

For some of the top tier endurance challenges (World's Toughest Mudder comes to mind), and certainly most of the classically designed ultra races (Western States 100, Leadville 100, that sort of thing) this ability to completely ignore the world and march to the beat of a single drum is an asset attained through countless hours running alone. However this trait is viewed as a critical flaw for many of the emerging and increasingly challenging endurance events where working with others is crucial for success.

Give me a gritty and determined team player happy with water and a Clif Bar over a vegan, soy milk sipping prima donna who has an aneurysm if his designer supplements are taken away any day. While that flake might have an insane mile split time, it was probably honed in ideal conditions to the beat of his favorite playlist. This kind of athlete will more than likely go to pieces faster than MRE pound cake when he is handed a forty pound water can that can't touch the ground and told to shoulder his portion of a 320 lb Zodiak watercraft for a five mile march up the beach.

In many of the more complex and team based endurance challenges that are rapidly gaining popularity over the traditional "one man shows" mule strength, a suicidal indifference to adversity, and the patience to shut the hell up at take all direction from the team leader are key traits. This ability makes the difference between a team that sails through every challenge posed to them and an argumentative hodgepodge circus wagon that earns the right to do everything the very hardest way possible all the live long day through to the end.

Being a team player is a crucial element for success in these events, but functioning well as a member of a team is not really something you can train for in a gym. Unfortunately, this fact often leaves people to think that altruism and team dynamics are completely hereditary and that their only choice is to wing it and hope for the best. Nothing could be further from the truth, the ability to get along with others can be honed and improved like a muscle in the body.

At its most philosophical, team work can be seen as a complex network of altruistic actions. People who have come together for a common end state and function together based on a series of 'I'll scratch your back if you scratch mine' interactions. Yes this does mean that teamwork is inherently somewhat selfish (there is hope for you marathoners). Each individual has to want to reach the goal, the issue is that the goal can't be reached alone so you have to help others so that they will help you back. The framework for teamwork has been established.

A crucial and refining point is personified in the old adage "Too many cooks in the kitchen spoil the broth." Concrete tasks with a hard and fast deadline need to be attacked. This means decisions need to be made fast and with conviction even if they are not the best overall solution (a bad decision is better than no decision).

What you cannot abide is an unstructured team with free flowing ideas.

A team leader needs to be established and everyone else needs to support that leadership completely. This means that when you are the leader you need to be confident and assertive and lead. When you are a follower you need to respect your ear to mouth ratio (listen twice as much as you speak) and support your leadership despite their shortcomings.

While the old saying "You are only as fast/strong and your slowest/weakest link" rings true it is mostly used as an insult hurled at failing team leaders or mumbled sarcastically when a task has been failed. An underlying lesson in leadership that is often glazed over when contemplating this element in team dynamics is the need for attentiveness and sympathy in a leader. A slow or weak link is not that much of a hindrance if handled quickly, effectively, and appropriately by an alert, mature, and attentive leader.

When your tire goes off the rim you are almost always better off stopping and calling AAA (mature, prepared, effective) than driving on that sucker 50 miles to the next service station in which case you may very well have utterly destroyed that part of your vehicle. In many instances it is simply not the best course of action to push through to completion given the situation. And in the case of intensely fatigued humans catch phrases and peppy one liners rarely get through let alone provide any kind of motivation.

In the same vein the approach of 'pushing harder until it works' rarely if ever does. So kicking a faltering member of the team along until mission completion is not going to win you any events. Most of the time a well timed pat on the back, a look in the eyes accompanied by a "Good work, keep it up buddy you've got this" is the difference between dead weight and a positive, contributing member of the team.

As a leader or battle buddy if you have the wherewithal to look around you then you are in good enough shape to notice and help others who are having trouble. Leave someone struggling to get deeper into their own head and flap in the wind and you will soon have serious issues to deal with. Or worse yet they will quit and you will have one less team member and just as much weight to carry.

One thing that team events teach you eventually is that life is not a spectator sport. I feel as though this lesson is going to become more and more important as our lives become increasingly remote and digitized. What I mean is that you quickly realize that the level that you involve yourself in the task at hand really does affect overall success and failure of your mission.

It is difficult for the human mind to grasp individual contribution in extremely large scale interactions like voting for a new president. But smaller scale efforts like hauling a super heavy pelican case for five miles with a group of ten people rotating in and out give an easy lesson in 'pulling your own weight'. You quickly figure out if you try to hang back and watch from the sidelines things really do happen slower and less effectively without you contributing.

"Getting lost in your own head" happens a lot in extreme endurance events and it can be the reason for a lot of DNF's. When severely stressed the mind has a tendency to focus inwards on all the pain and adversity you are facing. Overcoming this and gaining proper perspective (it could always be worse; I am still alive and moving) alone can be very hard.

The ones who can most easily do this are athletes with a lot of life experience and accumulated wisdom (why you see so many ultra endurance athletes over the age of 35). However, as a member of a proactive team it is easy (or should be at least) to get yourself out of your own head and help others do the same. Pay attention to your own thoughts and preoccupy yourself with the well being of your fellow teammates.

Especially in long and stressful events people will go through 'mood swings'. This stems from a multitude of different factors both internal and external. The short and sweet version of it is though that it is not safe or smart to write someone off as 'tough' or 'good to go' and ignore them after that. Everyone needs to be considered frequently as regrettable decisions are often made during momentary periods of weakness which can come on suddenly and with little warning. If you are a leader then watch your people and take care of them and if you are a team member then keep an eye on your battle buddy and don't be afraid to speak up if either of you are having a seriously rough time of it.

Lets explore the idea of 'battle buddy' for a minute. This is simply a slang term for person you look out for and care about intensely during a period of time. Their safety, accountability, and well being are just about as important to you as your own.

Necessarily they reciprocate this mentality and the two of you are bonded together in this fashion. I cannot tell you how many events I have been in that are technically 'individual' where I performed far better and more effectively because I latched onto another participant and we supported each other. If the event is academic in nature then you have a study buddy, and if it is physical then you have a partner to help out in the difficult stretches.

There are of course details to this kind of relationship that are delicate and as with all relationships, effective communication is key. If the event you are in is not inherently team based (meaning that you can finish the race independent of other participants) then you may want to come to some kind of mutual agreement ahead of time that you will split up if one member is beyond encouragement to keep up. You may however determine that finishing together is more important than your finishing time and decide to finish together no matter what. This is great, just make sure the other person is on the same page as you.

In other circumstances the finishing of the event is dependent on a team of participants making it together. In such a case the entire team can sometimes be disqualified if even one of the team members quits or is injured. In this type of scenario monitoring teammates for mood, injury, and motivation is nearly as important as performance. Here is where prior training as a team and the closeness of the teammates really pays for itself.

The more time the team has spent together before the event and the more they have trained for the chaos and rigours of the event the easier it will be to read each other's moods, physical state, and motivation at the time. This type of preparation will save significant amounts of time over a group who can't figure out if someone is really hurting or is just feeling bad for themselves. Attention still needs to be paid however, and a team that simply pushes as hard as possible for the fastest completion time is taking a huge risk of disqualification.

There is a subtle but substantial difference between someone who signs up for a team challenge unsure of whether or not they are completely prepared (there is no way to be 100% sure), and someone who comes in planning to depend on the team to get them through the event. Under ideal circumstances, when entering a team event you should prepare yourself to undertake the upcoming challenge alone. This will make the fact that you are part of a team an asset that makes tasks easier rather than a crutch you can use as an excuse to undertrain or show up unprepared.

Mental stress and fatigue are a somewhat special case because like physical stress and pain it cannot be garnered through much else but first hand experiences. The difference being that resilience to mental adversity is hard to train for in a gym. This is usually where the more experienced members of a team will have to step up and support newer members who whilst being physically sound, have not figured out their mental weaknesses and associated coping mechanisms. It should be said however that generally the more physically strong you are going into the challenge the longer you can stave off mental stress and destructive feelings.

Sometimes however, it can be hard to tell what kind (mental or physical) of issues a team member is dealing with. Being able to read a fellow teammate and help them out of their slump is an essential skill and the sign of a proactive veteran of team based challenges. It is an exercise in reason and wisdom to understand that when the team needs to finish together the state of each member of that team cannot be ignored or bludgeoned away through insults or half hearted platitudes. When a single member breaks down and thereby slows down the entire effort, it is an equal failure on the part of the team for allowing that person to go that far down that dark road. Seasoned team endurance challenge athlete Mark Webb discusses this team dynamic:

"During the event, someone enters the darkness of their mind, demons are hitting hard, and they hate life. This is possibly the hardest thing they have done and may not have developed the mental tools yet to overcome that and turn the scenario around. Therefore if you KNOW how to overcome demons you should instead be eagerly doing all you can to help that "sufferer" (sometimes called sandbagger) out of their hell pit and into the light.

There are a gazillion ways to do this. You can start telling jokes, ask them about themselves and get them talking, start a chant, or even just look at them and tell them to smile. Sometimes saying "I know you are hurting, but can you take this weight for just one block" is enough to bring someone back. A few words, a few distractions are often all it takes to turn someone from a suffering individual on a team to a hard working teammate.

So to reiterate, if you feel a sandbagger didn't deserve their patch then perhaps you don't deserve it for failing to motivate them when they needed your help in their darkest hour. They may have done less but I guarantee they suffered more."

This can often happen in less intense events where there is a mixture of very experienced and very new participants. In the worst cases the veterans will form an exclusive group and shut out the newer participants and leave them to their fate. While the new participants may be capable of solving the challenges presented there is still a schism in the group as a whole and by definition tasks or challenges cannot be solved or overcome as efficiently as they possibly could.

What about events that actively discourage working together? There are a few of the hardest endurance competitions where event officials work towards keeping participants separated, silent, and unable to help other participants. In such circumstances fellow participants can still help each other out albeit in an indirect and dark manner.

By 'zooming out' of the incredibly arduous task you are being told to execute and seeing other people around you doing the same thing you can help jar your mind back into perspective. This will reassure your mind that the task at hand is indeed possible to complete because there are other humans around you doing just that! And in the less uncommon than you might think event that you are the only participant left in the event you can gather strength from the fact that you are the strongest person there and that you now have to prove that you alone have the strength to persevere and make it to the end of the event.

Something else you see in high level endurance challenges that can be tricky to navigate is remote team forming. Events like Death Race and World's Toughest Mudder have options for teams to enter and participate together. However because elite athletes able to make good placements in these events are few and far between, it is not uncommon for teams to be formed of individuals from all corners of the country or world.

For those of you hoping to break into these top tier events as part of team to make things a little easier and have more support you may find trouble with this approach. Unless you have three to five friends with identical athletic aspirations and five hundred plus dollars to blow you will likely have to try to apply to an existing team. If this is the case then I hope you have been social at previous events and made some friends along with having attained some respectable achievements because you are going to need them now.

As with many ultra endurance sports the field of frequent competitors is small. Especially for newer categories like endurance challenges. Everyone knows everyone here and so getting onto a team can have a lot to do with who you know and how much they like you. If you are contacting the guy who saw you quit at the last big event because you had a boo boo on your foot I would not expect a call back.

In the unlikely event that the potential team members do not know each other they will likely use performance at a previous event as a benchmark for determining the ability level of the petitioning athletes. Again, past performance reflects on future prospects so be sure to give it everything you've got even if the event you are in is not your 'ultimate goal', your potential future teammates are watching. And as with other situations in life, getting in can be as much about who you know as what you know so realise that someone might be staking their reputation on your giving a strong performance for the team.

The unexpected can cause an athlete to get thrown off their stride with depressing ease. For both events that are individually run or participated in as part of a team (competitive or noncompetitive) the ability to be unperturbed by the unexpected and to be able to adapt quickly and efficiently to novel situations is an essential skill for success. Ultra endurance athlete Olof Dallner faced a truck load of novel situations and unexpected stresses during his Quintuple IRONMAN.

Though not a competitive event (each athlete was just tasked with finishing) accountability nevertheless came into play not only in dealing with his personal situation but with his interaction with others on the course. Critical decisions were made that greatly affected the success or failure of the participants. Mistakes were made but the adaptability and level headedness of Olof and his fellow participants allowed things to get back on a reasonable track quickly enough to salvage the situation and facilitate a strong finish. In his words:

"There are a couple of things that changed the way this race went down. First, just a few days before it looked like the weather would be great. That suddenly changed. At lunch time the second day it started pouring down and it was continuous rain from then to the finish. The weather made it a lot harder to keep your pace up. Second, I had a planned pace to keep for my run. That changed when for some reason me and Andy started racing. We had several almost sprints when we wanted to knock the air out of each other.

About halfway in, after 70 miles or so, I think we did 10 miles at a 8min/mile pace. We crashed after that and had to spend some time recovering. It was very stupid and I'm not sure why we did that, it would've cost us our finish. We actually shook hands out on the course and agreed to stop doing that and finish together instead. I sat down for a while to wait for Andy to catch up to me and then we went together. However, our sprints had taken a toll on Andy's ankles, he could not run anymore. So we split up again and I pushed forward."

The self examination and critical reasoning under immense stress required to assess a faulty approach and return to a state of maximum civility in this situation was impressive. Both athletes realized that they had been mistaken in getting overly competitive with each other and that this course of action was actively decreasing the chances of either of them finishing the event. With competitive tactics not conducive to the ability to finish or overall standing they were smart and focused on what was actually important for the event at hand. Losing sight of what the real objectives for your event are can not only cost you time, effort, and post event friends, it can cost you the event itself.

Some Extra Stories

Tieing together a little bit of all the topic areas we have covered so far, James Vreeland's recounting of his experiences at Peak Race's 2014 Winter Death Race is a gem I want to provide for you uncut and in its entirety. The Death Race is known for being unpredictable, grueling, long, and frustrating as hell. Mind games play almost as much a part of this event as the physical challenges do. To make it through this top tier endurance challenge a participant needs to be physically and mentally tough. But unlike a more cookie cutter event, participants need to be flexible and adaptable to constantly changing and chaotic situations as the race is never the same year to year.

Winter Death Race 2014

JAMES VREELAND

Pre race directions were that the event would begin at 3pm, sharp. We were instructed to drop our gear in the lower level of the brown barn (any time between noon and 3pm) and be ready for race briefing at 2:50pm. Upon arriving at the barn around 12:45pm, there was no one present, we dropped gear and made our way to the General Store and met up with other racers.

Posted in the store was a note stating "good wages offered to anyone who wished to split wood prior to the race", along with a contact number and directions to apply in person at Amee Farms. At this point we all began playing "Death Race Chicken", we were obviously going to end up splitting logs, but arrive too early and you were likely to simply add time to your workload. Showing up late would be bad as well. The racers I was with elected to arrive about an hour early and just accept the possibility of some extra work. This was the first of several well constructed mind games.

On arriving at Amee Farms in response to the help wanted ad, racers were informed that there was a change in the rules. This year's Death Race was only open to legal employees of the state of Vermont. We however were in luck, as we could apply as independent contractors to split logs for $1 an hour. Immediately my hopes of actually making it back to the barn for an on-time start went out the window, and I started splitting. Over time more racers streamed in and started working for permission to start their race.

Around 3pm we heard staff radios crackle to life as Joe starting berating the lack of attention to detail from the attendees and informed volunteers that several racers (who had shown up early to split timber) were already registered and the race had begun. 90% of the field was already behind. A few hours later (depending on when you arrived to the farm) we were paid for our services and told to report to the barn for registration.

side note: I can't wait to get a 1099-MISC tax form for $5 around this time next year

At the barn we were scolded for screwing up already. There was a schedule to be kept, and most of us had missed the first event (a time trial hike, under load). We lined up for registration, only to find out that the price of the race had also increased by $5. There went my newly found lumberjack wealth. During registration we were informed of the final rules for the race. Each racer would be collecting pieces of a puzzle, first person to complete their puzzle wins the race. Completing events would earn you another piece of the puzzle. Racers who started on-time were completing their ruck, new racers could not start this event because we had a mandatory meeting at the barn in ~an hour. Normally, the first day or so of the Death Race is mostly group tasks - this time, the actual "race" portion started immediately.

At the appointed time, we were introduced to local

guides who would be schooling us in the arts of starting fires and not freezing to death. Teams of two (you had to find yourself a partner before the event) went about the task of creating batches of char cloth and practiced building fires using flint and steel. February in Vermont is cold and wet, dry tinder sources are not very abundant.

Once everyone had done a reasonably poor job of preparing ourselves for backwoods survival, we were told to gear up with minimal packs, and the group trekked over to Amee Farms. The pace was quick, the trail already dark, and the group rapidly spread out. As we filtered in, we were instructed to drop our gear on the lower level and strip down to "dancing clothes". Things just got a little sexier. For the next 4 or so hours Eileen led us through remedial ballet lessons in a rocket-hot upper room.

At some point, Joe decided that we were having too much fun and figured that he had seen enough ballet to make up some new moves/exercises for us to try. 500 toe kicks per leg, go. 15 minutes of balancing on one foot with your arms held out, do it. Joe's recital carried on for quite some time, a few people got pulled outside to do burpees because staff didn't like their form, or they were smiling, or some other petty offense. Finally we were done and instructed to gear up and hustle back to the barn, with a hard time cutoff. Everyone put the hammer down and fast marched through the blackness.

Back at camp we received a puzzle piece and were told that we had until 5am to accumulate laps up and down the mountain to try to rack up puzzle pieces. First lap was with your full gear, second lap with a lighter pack, alternate, lather, rinse, repeat. No one could start a lap after 3:30am because we had another group task starting then. Every "odd" numbered trip we had to carry the worst part of our packing list - a 70lb tube of sand. For most racers, adding this item brought your pack weight to right around 100lbs. Our route up the mountain was around a mile each way, up set after set of stone stairs, in the dark, covered in ice, while snowing. You simply had to get from basecamp to Joe's cabin, check in, turn yourself around, and head down the slope.

Sure footing was not guaranteed, and a number of racers bowed out of the event on their first lap. A few lead racers made it back from their third lap (second with full weight) in time to fit in a "quick" jog up and back to score 4 puzzle pieces during the night. I finished three laps and took a few minutes at the barn to swap out socks and a base layer, having missed the 3:30am cutoff for additional laps by 15-20 minutes.

All active racers having now come down off the mountain, we were tasked with building a fire (no matches/chemical aids) with our partner. The flames had to exceed the markings on some arbitrary measuring stick (about 3' tall) for 3 or 5 seconds, then you could collect another piece. A quick and (for most) easy prize. This is where a little extra planning paid off, I had stashed dry tinder after our initial fire building activities and had a decent supply of dryer lint tucked in to my kit bag. Sparks became flames, flames became a puzzle piece.

We were then told to prep to be far away from basecamp for an extended period of time, at least 4-6 hours. After jocking up, we set off towards Sable Mountain. To collect this task, we had to make our way to the foot of the mountain, check in, ascend to the summit, check in, return to base, check in, and return to basecamp. This turned out to be our longest movement of the challenge at around 15 miles round trip. The first half of the trek to Sable was through familiar trails. Lots of switchbacks and steep icy ascents, after which we moved to dirt roads and you could pick up the pace.

It was really beginning to feel like a race. At the base of the mountain, racers were told that they had to complete a total of 100 burpees before they could head back to camp. Some people did 50 before their ascent, 50 after descending. I elected to just get them out of the way and banged out a pretty quick 100 then set off up the slope. The sun was just starting to come up and it was refreshing to see new terrain, so the majority of the ascent was quite nice. There were a few false summits that caused a little internal sighing, but moving forward quickly put those issues behind you.

The final pitch to the summit of Sable Mountain is quite steep and groups bunched up on the trail. There was a little jockeying for position to break away from the packs, but most people knew there were many miles ahead of us and no one lost their cool. The summit itself was tree-covered and didn't have good visibility (bummer), but after checking in/turning around you encountered some stunning views of early morning light on the way down. Incredibly gorgeous, when you could take your eyes off the trail plummeting away ahead of you.

This was the first time you could gauge the other racers as you passed each other on the way up/down. Some people were hurting, but for the most part, the remaining group was doing well. I checked in at the base, where they verified that my 100 burpees were done, and headed down the long dirt road home, having some great conversations with other racers along the way. My out and back took right around 5 hours.

Back at basecamp, the leaders (who had finished their time trial ruck the day before) headed off in one direction. The rest of us "got" the chance to make up that timed event now. Yippie. Our big old bag of sand was loaded in to our gear, and we were given a loop to follow up the the summit of Joe's Mountain.

With fresh legs, and skill in the mountains, the leaders made this loop in ~1:45 the day before. I was now targeting anything under 3 hours. There are a lot of heavy ruck miles in my background, and they served me well here. I passed/caught quite a few racers on this segment and completed my loop is around 2:20. Along the way, we saw the leaders excitedly carrying their sandbags, dropping hints that they were on their way to get rid of that burden during the next event. Spirits were raised a hair.

At the barn we were told that we had until a specific time (5 or 6pm, I think) to complete our next two tasks, or we would be dropped. Failing this wasn't an option (though, knowing this race, that cutoff could easily have been a lie). Next up: "Go see Joe at Amee Farms, take your sandbag". A quick hike later we learned that we then had to hold our sandbags (70lbs) overhead for 45 minutes. Whiskey Tango F-this. Tasks, however, are non-negotiable, so the bags went up. Luckily you could rest the weight on your head, so the work was painful, but doable. As my clock counted down to zero, I worked my way over to the pile of dumped sandbags and prepped to get rid of that heavy SOB. My neck and shoulders have rarely felt as good as they did after throwing that weight away. Back to the barn.

Our next chore was to report to Peter's house, and expect to be hanging out for a while. This should be interesting. Over the hill and through the woods to Peter's house we went. First thing you noticed were big piggy banks spray painted on to the snow. The second thing you noticed were people with a hand ziptied to their foot digging through the ice and slush. Turns out that months ago the children of the area had scattered pennies all over the yard, then it snowed.

We had to collect 30 pennies and count them out into the piggy bank before we could cut our zip tie and leave. There were a few tricks on how to find pennies, but for the most part, it was hunting and pecking and digging around in the snow. If you broke your zip tie bond early, you lost all of your current stash and had to do somersaults. Sitting on your butt in the snow put a good chill in to the bones, but my partner from earlier (Mark Webb) struck gold and we were out of there in a pretty reasonable time. We had heard whispers that the race was about to turn masochistic, but figured that that was either idle chatter, or part of HQ's plan to get into our heads. We were wrong.

In any event like this, the thing that keeps me going is the knowledge that no matter how bad your current task is, eventually it will end and you will do something different. That new thing might be better or worse, but it will be new. That little change in modality is a godsend. At this point I had 9 out of what appeared to be a 24 piece puzzle, and we were ~26 hours into the race. I refused to do the mental math to estimate remaining time, but knew it wasn't in my favor.

Checking in at basecamp brought some unwelcome news. The remainder of the race was really simple: Ascend Joe's mountain, check in, return to base, get a piece. After every round you had the option to build another fire (on your own) for an additional piece. I had 15 pieces left to collect; this was going to be a long night.

My fire-making skills were pretty solid, so it was faster for me to take the time at basecamp to scrounge wood and build a fire for the extra piece (even though it meant sitting still and getting cold). Some people couldn't make a spark to save their life, but were mountain goats, so they opted out of the fire tasks and simply hiked laps to chip away at their remaining pieces.

By the time I got back to basecamp, the leaders had really separated from the pack - getting their time trials out of the way the day before, scoring a fourth ascent last night (before our trip to Sable), and getting to the Penny Farm while most of the field had to make up their time trial meant the top places were already locked up. Coming in, my goal was simply to finish, but I still wanted to do well. I was at least 6 pieces behind 1st as I started my hill cycles.

This task took forever. I come from the Midwest, we don't have mountains. All of this aggressive hill climbing was taking its toll. I was fading. Periodically we were given updates of you must have XX pieces by XX:XX to stay in the race. I didn't have to sprint, but I couldn't screw around and take long breaks if I wanted to stay ahead of the cuts. My lowest points of the race happened in the coming hours. I wasn't as on top of my nutrition as I should have been, and I bonked often.

My saving grace was that I could turn my brain off and put one foot in front of the other throughout the night. Then the snow started, and the trail became harder to follow. At the summit a few crafty souls found a bail of dry hay to make fire-starting easier down the trail. Thick, wet snow blanketed everything, making tinder almost impossible to source. People's nerves were fraying and guttural cries were common.

Finally, while checking in with the ladies at basecamp, I got a weird look from the lovely soul passing out puzzle pieces. I only had a few left. My final tasks were to build two fires (because I had an odd number of pieces left), ascend the mountain one final time, and assemble my puzzle. I could walk up there one more time. Easy day, all day. I was physically spent, but mentally in a good place, so I took my time climbing this final time, stopping a few times along the way to reflect on the race. I knew the time cutoffs, and where I stood. I was going to take some "me" time, and in retrospect, I'm glad I did - it brought a nice close to the event for me. With my puzzle built, I started my descent to camp with a delirious smile on my face.

At camp, I checked in, got my skull, took a few photos, thanked all of the volunteers (Seriously, they are the best. All of us racers are deeply indebted to them for their service), and promptly spaced out. My group still had racers on the course, so I stuck around for a while policing my gear, tending to my feet, and eating half a sheet pan of leftover catering that the volunteers were done with. With every person that came in off the course, we cheered, passed around half drank celebration beers, and helped them shed gear. It was a unique experience that so little fanfare followed such a large event, but it felt quite fitting and I loved it.

With all of my team off the mountain and the event officially capped, we loaded in to cars and made our way to a B&B where I brushed my teeth and fell asleep in the corner almost immediately. That next morning, we rose and grabbed first and second breakfast at the B&B before making our way back to the General Store for one of their world famous egg sandwiches. I had heard about them previously, but assumed their praise was at least partially hyperbole from famished racers. It was not. That sandwich made the entire ordeal worthwhile; the heavens opened up and placed ham and egg on brioche, then delivered it to my log table with a large side of hot sauce, and it was good.

All said and done racers completed: 65 miles of travel (around 10-15 of that under the full sandbag load), 40k feet of elevation gain, and up to 36 hours of racing.

James's experiences and methodology for dealing with the challenges he faced reflect numerous points made so far in this work.

Making the Challenge more of a 'challenge'

We can learn a lot about an upcoming challenge by speaking with people who have already been through it. Sharing experiences is one of our species strongest uses of the beautiful tool that is language. In my opinion not asking as many intelligent questions as possible before showing up for a major event is setting yourself at a needless disadvantage (maybe that is something you are into but I personally am not). People who thrive in these endurance challenges also tend to be type A personalities more than happy to regale you with every detail of their experience.

Todd Kruse is one such Type A motivated individual who has made a hobby of crushing the grueling ten to twelve hour Goruck Challenge over and over again. This is a team event involving carrying heavy and awkward loads through water, sand, and city streets at the direction of a current or former SOF soldier. They are no joke and no two Challenges are ever the same. To make things even harder on himself Todd decided to do two of them 'Back to Back' with only a few hours break in between. Enjoy his story and learn from it if you ever intend to tackle the Challenge some day, and if you're already a GRT then you'll sympathize with much of Todd's story.

No matter your fitness level or past experiences, your first GORUCK Challenge is always something at least a little special and always memorable. That is just the nature of the set up. Even if you are a physical specimen who can crush the demanding standard set by the cadre you will still be forced to mentally adapt to changing situations and do so in the company of new and diverse teammates. This is what makes the GORUCK Challenge so much more than other endurance events; teamwork and problem solving are not optional.

With that said, it is possible to become 'good' at GORUCK Challenges. Even though you are being led by masters of chaos, if you stick with it you eventually start speaking the language. This started becoming the case for a few diehards in the GORUCK community who started racking up Tough patches in the double digits.

These were people who loved the event, the atmosphere, and the people, but just wanted MORE! Enter the back to back Challenge, more simply known as B2B. Because GORUCK cadre tend to do two iterations on a given weekend (typically Friday night and Saturday night) rucktards realized that they could make it to both (with a couple hours in between classes). And so begins the story of the B2B Challenge; for those who want their 'Two Scoops' of Good Livin'.

Silly Man

By: Todd 'Patches' Kruse

I had decided that I wanted to do a back to back challenge in Charlotte. This was February sixteenth 2013 and would consist of classes 413 and 420. At first it was because I had friends who were doing both classes and couldn't get together to do a single class as a group. The second reason came out of wanting to test myself to see if I could do this, with the reasoning that if I could then I MIGHT just make it through half of a Selection class. That was pure shit, but training motivation nonetheless. After talking with Kovak and Cadre Dan, they said that doing B2B wouldn't do anything for me as far as Selection was concerned. So, what the hell...let's do a back 2 back anyway.

With about a month before the Challenge date, I had been rucking once a week early Saturday morning with some of my future classmates. It was cold, dark and sucked... I figured; perfect warm up for the Challenge. The chatter on the Goruck Tough page started to pick up, and people noticed I was doing both classes. One of these people was Cadre Rich who would be one of the cadre present during that weekend. He asked if I was really signed up for both. I said yes, and he replied back with two simple words: "Silly Man"

Silly Man...Don't know what he was thinking those words would do to me. But one thing I don't do is back down from a challenge. "CHALLENGE ACCEPTED". I was going to do both classes, I was going to smile through all the shit, and at the end of it, show myself how silly I really am.

Challenge night, 0100 2/16/2013 Class 413:

I got to the start location with a CRV (I know, sexy) full with my ruck, two flags with flag poles (learned my lesson from class 192) and a team weight. A NASCAR "tire" with heavy metal chains screwed into it for added weight and easier carrying. I walked down to the start with items in tow only to see that Cadre Dan and Cadre Bert were there with a shit ton of stuff already. Two eighty pound slosh pipes, three twenty five pound water jugs, the Pittsburgh Steel team weight, a kit bag, and a few other items. And then there was the long-ass rope festooned carabineers.

When cadre was ready to take roll call, there were only twelve of us standing there. Dan is not happy. There were originally eighteen people signed up and so he had brought a corresponding amount of coupons to carry (AKA a Shit-ton). He kept telling us: "You had better hope more people show up or you are all going to hate life". The other six never did, so roll call it was. There wasn't a welcome party at the start point, but we knew it was coming. The police showed up and I think they wanted us to move. So we all attached ourselves to the rope supplied to us by the US Government and we headed out on our first mission.

"Get to Veterans Park" - Time Hack 1 hour

I had no clue where Veterans Park was which made

me glad I wasn't the team leader. But, we had a few people who knew the area well, and Dan was generous on the first mission by showing us the location on his phone, which also gave us a sense of the distance we needed to cover. One hour was NOT going to be fun. We busted our ass, lots of fast walking, jaywalking and some light run/shuffles. We ran into a few "ladies of the night" but politely declined services and just kept going. We made it up the park entrance and found that we had made the hack by two minutes and were rewarded with a twenty minute break. What happened next was a shit ton of fun, and by that I mean a world of suck.

We unhooked from the rope and dropped all team weights and moved to home base on a baseball diamond. We then proceeded to do "He's up, he sees me, I'm down" drills (buddy team rushes) for 400-500 yards back and forth across the baseball diamond. Then we repeated the drill but with a team casualty and low crawling (serious

Motivation for Current and Aspiring Endurance Challenge Athletes

suck). Then the same again but with TWO casualties (more suck). Then fireman carries, relay runs, etc. By the time that was finished, no one was cold, everyone was sweating and tired. Dan had us sit and told us WHY we did all those things, as Dan is often inclined to do.

"Get to Park Road Park" - Time Hack 2 hours

FUCK ME! From Veterans Park to Park Road Park is pretty much from one side of the city to the other. We hooked up, grabbed our gear and headed out. Just then we received the first bad news of the night. One of my teammates notices that my water bladder is leaking, my back is all wet! I tried to check the bladder, it seemed fine, but I'm still leaking water; I resign myself to check this after it's all done, have to keep moving! After some back tracking, and taking side streets we got to a location that I actually knew and could point out on a map. I had a clear route planned for the TL. But, my plan was vetoed and we took more side streets. Guess what...we got lost. It was at this point, around 3:30am that it started to rain. I was wet, started to get cold and really didn't like it.

This was the first and only time during either of the challenges that weekend that I thought about quitting. Jen will tell you...rain sucks, especially when the temperature is just above freezing. The navigator kept telling us what we would be seeing our objective around the next corner... but it never seemed to materialize. We get out to a Park Road and I realize we are almost 2 miles off course! Needless to say, we missed the time hack. We rolled into Park Road Park and headed to a covered picnic area. We were right next to a lake...

Miss a time hack, you get punished.

The sun is now up, Dan looks happy, actually smiling and giggling I think. He says:"hrmm a lake, and you missed your time hack, wonder if I planned this? Yeah, I did."He gives us two minutes to take off anything we don't want to get wet. Shoes have to stay on, rucksacks come with us. Two guys approach Dan wanting to quit, they are talked back into sticking around. We march to the water.

No shit, this water was cold! But something strange happened... I didn't give a fuck. I started smiling, even laughing; I think it pissed cadre off. We went out to mid thigh, and did squats with rucks over head. I'm making noises and smiling. We finished in the water, and were told to lose the rope, coil it up and stuff it in the kit bag. Time for our next mission.

"Get to Bank of America Stadium"- No Time Hack Given

I am selected to be team leader for this one. I construct a clear route in my head and we step off. I'm in good spirits, but not sure about everyone else. I doubt there was a single smile between us. Why you may ask? It may have been the sleet/snow that was now falling continuously. But we pressed on regardless. I'm going up and down the lines making sure everyone was OK, etc etc, and trying to scrape together some motivation. The "navigator" then claims he has a faster way to get there so we take a detour off of my original route. I get pulled

Motivation for Current and Aspiring Endurance Challenge Athletes

aside by Bert and told that I now had one hour to get there. One hour to go 6-7 miles. No fucking way that is going to happen. I relay this to the team and one of them jokingly says "Hey, let's take the train!" Bert hears this and says "You will burn for it if you do". But remembering back to Dan's speech that he gave us at the beginning: "If you ain't cheatin', you ain't tryin" Or "Work with the grey areas". We approach the main street where the train runs and two of the team decide they have had enough. They disappear.

At this point, we get punished for taking the train, or we get punished for missing our new time hack. I give in, and agree that we should take the train. We get to the train platform and someone graciously coughs up the 20 bucks for everyone to ride. Dan asks what we are doing, I said "taking the train". He asks why, I tell him "We need to get creative." No answer from Dan, so I figure we aren't too far off base. We make it to the bank, missing our time hack AND taking the train. Find out we are the ONLY GRC team to use mass transit. Point of pride I guess. As we get to the Stadium, Bert informs us that we get to go out onto the field. It's been prearranged...very cool. But since we were a half hour late, we have to haul ass. We get on the field, and take a few pictures. I give my class patch to Bert to give to our gracious host as a thank you. And off we go.

"Get to the NASCAR Hall of Fame": - Time Hack 25 minutes(?)

We calculate that our objective should only be about seven blocks from our current location. We were looking good to finally make a time hack! Off we go! We move as fast as we can until we are within less than a block from the objective when Dan stops us and asks how many people are in our class. Shit! In the back of my mind I know what is coming next. Someone had dropped back or was snatched up by the cadre and we hadn't seen it! Time for some punishment; push-ups, flutter kicks, etc which then subsequently caused us to miss our time hack...again.

But we got some good photo opportunities in front of the NASCAR hall of fame so it wasn't a total morale killer.

"Get back to Freedom Park" - Time Hack 1.5 hours

Did they say Freedom Park? THAT'S WHERE WE STARTED! Holy SHIT! Could this be the end? We get about four different opinions as to how to get back there. I suggested that we take the Greenway (essentially a pedestrian walkway that winds its way through the park at one point), others give different route suggestions. I get a little frustrated at this point. I'm tired; I have taken this route there before (see during GRC 192 in Charlotte the previous year). The collective mind eventually decides on a different route. We get down to where the Greenway starts and it becomes quickly obvious that taking it will be much easier...they switch back to my route suggestion. We take it, and get to the park with plenty of time left. Time hack beat!

Done...or are we?

Nope, not even close! Remember that smoke session at the beginning? Oh wait, we didn't have one...It's on, NOW.

We do a bunch of "fun" drills and we also get a very small taste of a favorite SFAS event: Log PT (a cadre Dan personal favorite). But first we had to FIND the logs. After getting logs we commence log PT for what I'm guessing is a fraction of the time SFAS classes are put through, despite this, it is still a severe smoke session; I fear my arms are going to fall off. A few more drills and then Dan tags Cadre Bert in to give us a second scoop of good livin'. Cadre Bert is fair, and believes in rewards for good behavior and punishment for missing things. FAIR! So, since he is a strong believer in knowing your team, he gives us a chancy but reachable objective. Two people, in a row, need to name every team member by first name only, and we are done. Miss a name, we get punished. Sadly, this takes a few rounds of pain and agony. With me failing miserably right off the bat. Push-ups, flutter kicks oh crap! PT sessions have a way of jogging memories and soon enough we get two people in a row who can meet the task and we are now officially DONE!

Patches are handed out; beers are enjoyed and talk of tonight's 2200 class starts.

Oh yeah, and that leaky water bladder? It was actually a beer that had become a casualty from all the fun at Veterans Park so now my pack smells of beer, mmmmm.

Guess I better get home and rest up. According to the weather reports it's going to be a lot colder tonight, and all my stuff is wet. And I need to eat!

Let's do this thing!

Challenge Night, 2200 2/16/2013 Class 420:

I had gotten about 5 hours of good sleep, a ton of food and my clothes dried. I didn't bother washing them...what's the point? A fellow classmate was kind enough to come pick me up so I wouldn't have to drive to the start point or home (Figuring I would be completely out of it afterwards, which I was!). So Cheers to Mark! We get to the start point and haul down the team weights to the start point, flags, poles, etc. Feels like I've done this before.

Tonight is Cadre Bert's turn to shine in his inaugural Goruck Class with Cadre Dan shadowing to make sure all is right during the challenge (New cadre do a GRC, then shadow a GRC, the lead a GRC, often one right after another before becoming recognized as full cadre). Initially I thought I would see a completely different start to this challenge, I soon found out how wrong I was. What was lying there at the start point? All the same crap as last night! Slosh pipes, water jugs, old team weight, etc and that DAMN ROPE! We fall in for the scare brief (what to expect, short intros from our beloved cadre and a preview of the misery that lies ahead). Bert calls attention to me as having done the class last night, and to look to me for any help or hints on how to survive tonight. We find out our class number is 420. Bert decides to call us the "Pot Heads" all night. We love it.

Great, thanks Bert. Bert asks me what he feels to be very important. Without even thinking I shout out "NAMES!" I am correct; he tells us that we have ten minutes to learn everyone's names, all eighteen names. We get in a circle and start going around, again, again, and again. Despite this, I still have NO CLUE what everyone's names are. Our ten minutes are up and we get back in line. Bert repeats his mantra of "I'm a fair guy" and says that if we can get two people to go all the way down the line, in a row and nail all the first names, we move out, no punishment. My mind flashes back to last night and how many rounds of PT it took to get this right. The first guy steps out and NAILS it! Holy shit! This might just be our night! The second guy comes out and launches into the names and gets about three fourths of the way down and stalls...holy shit...a few seconds later, the light goes on in his head and he finishes up the names. TWO IN A ROW! The entire class is screaming and cheering; we dodged some punishment right out of the gate! Bert is VERY impressed. So, being a fair guy, we step off.

"Get to Latta Park" - Time Hack 25 minutes

I was selected to be the first team leader; I asked around if anyone knew where the park was. Nobody had a clue, nada, nothing. SHIT. Bert is trying to drop hints behind me and I'm getting the sense that it must be close. So we step off, figure we can figure it out on the way. We head out just as the police show up at the start point. As we move past businesses I start looking for people outside bars, etc. I find a guy and ask him where the park is, he says it's up a ways and turn right. I thank him and we keep going. Using his directions we arrive at the park well ahead of the Time Hack. It pays to ask for directions! Nicely done class and I am promptly fired. Reward: ten minutes to rehydrate and to keep quiet.

"Get to Veterans Park" - Time Hack 1 hour 30 minutes

New team leader and a new mission... Knowing the park' location from the previous night's Challenge I get the location and directions to the TL and step back into line and snap into the "dog leash" as it's now being called. Our TL was amazing. He knew we had a very hard time hack. Honestly, I doubted from the start that we were going to make it. But, he had us shuffle for a block or two, slow to a fast walk, and kept us motivated. Team weights were passed around, everyone getting to hold something for a few minutes while someone else rested. It's a party night in Charlotte, all the bars are hoping and we find ourselves yelling "GORUCK!" quite often to people drunkenly yelling after us as to what we are doing. The TL is asking me if we are close, and I'm doing my best as guessing distance. We get close and tell him. We start shuffling fast; despite this I still think we missed the time hack. We get to the park and find out we CRUSHED the time hack with over four minutes to spare! Everyone is thrilled! Two for two! Reward: twenty minutes to rest, stuff some food down, pee, and rehydrate.

Special Mission: "Beat Cadre Patrick's Class to the Memorial Statue" - Time Hack ASAP

Motivation for Current and Aspiring Endurance Challenge Athletes

We pick up a new TL and since we were at the park, I thought we were going to have some 'fun' getting smoked like the previous night's class with buddy carries, buddy team rushes, etc. Nope! Different mission, something different this time. Remember F3? You don't, ask someone from 192. In short, we don't like them. It turns out that Cadre Patrick is leading the F3 folks. All 80 of them; you heard me, 80! He has I believe two other cadre supporting him. But our mission now is to beat the F3 folks to a memorial statue. And we hear yet again "It pays to be a winner!" New TL in the lead, two time hacks crushed, lets rock and roll.

We head out, walking fast and shuffling on and off. We get closer to the objective (still not in sight) and Bert gets a text from Patrick. F3 is lost; SWEET! We are about 200 yards from the statue when we see it. Patrick is there; he lied. Result, we lose and Bert is not happy. The F3 group is doing exercises...why? I have no clue. Bert then proceeds to smoke us pretty good. Pushups with team weights, flutter kicks with team weights, etc. and Patrick standing over us the whole time telling us how shitty we are. All of this in the snow as well = good livin' for everyone. After the smoke session, Bert gathers us around and gives us a small pep talk. The F3 group only had their required team weight and some water jugs. We had hundreds of pounds in other coupons on top of that and a fraction of the people. Not a full excuse by any means, but to be proud of what we did. Thanks Bert. This is also the time we start to see some people in the class start to not look so good. One guy is trying to make himself puke. Yum! We get a few minutes, but then it's time to move on.

"Get to Discovery Place" - Time Hack 1 hour

New TL and a new course set. I point the TL back towards uptown and we set off. Point of interest here for class 192 people. We went right by the gas station where we stopped for a break. Always smile when I see that place and think of you all.

Now we have two people that are puking up their

dinner. It's time for us to stop and wait to see if they can get better. Tick tock, tick tock...no rest for the wicked. Our time hack is slipping away, but we have to help our teammates who are not able to move and that's more important. We start off again eventually and it's not long before the cadre stops us. We lost a team member and didn't stop for him. Great...punishment at some point. We move him to the front so we can watch him and we keep going. Not feeling like we are going to make it, we arrive at Discovery Place and Bert asks the TL if we made the time hack. The TL responds with the rest of the team "No". Bert shows us the clock. We made it with two minutes to spare. So far three for three on time hacks!

Time for Punishment

In the heart of downtown Charlotte we were given the option to receive our punishment now or at the end of the challenge. We decide to take it now. Smoked doesn't even start to describe what were after this ordeal. It was about 45 straight minutes of fireman carries, push ups, flutter kicks, over head presses, relay races with rucks...At one point we do get a piece of funny news; it turns out someone called the cops, thinking that an "Occupy Charlotte" group was protesting in uptown. HA! After the punishment is dealt out, we get 10 minutes to rest and pull ourselves back together. We hit a bit of a low in morale, rest is no fun now as the temperature is consistently in the low twenties and the wind is horrible. We see three of our teammates quit and pile into a car, just like that. Now we are down to 15.

"Get to Panther Stadium" - Time Hack 30 Minutes

New TL (Alex Bradshaw) and she rocks it, we get there in plenty of time and take some fun pictures around the statues and chill for a few minutes.

"Get to the NASCAR Hall of Fame" - Time Hack 20 Minutes

Stepping off, Bradshaw is still team leader; we head to the NASCAR HOF. We reach it in time, but the cadre pulls us off the street and into the underground HEATED parking deck of the facility (we were told the wind chill had taken the temperature down to a balmy five degrees ... Flipping cold!). Ah heat, wonderful! We get about ten minutes to rest and warm up a little. But as Bert says, with a reward comes a cost.

The price is no fun (but still worth it). Starting with elephant walks in a circle until we can do it in step and in time for 30 seconds which that takes us a few minutes to get down correctly, but we finish it and faster than expected. Next, we head to the ramp going down to the next level, we line up in one line across the space and bear crawl down to the next level, then as a group in a line holding bags, we sprint to the other end of the flat level, then we repeat this alternating of exercises all the way down to the bottom floor of the garage. The heat from the ramp now feels like a punishment, everyone is sweating and constantly drinking their water. We switched up from bear crawls to elephant walks down the ramps, not much better but a little tolerable. We are now at the bottom and receive our next mission.

"Get to Dunkin Donuts" - Time Hack 25 Minutes

The group has to get itself to a Dunkin Donuts close to the Greenway. I know where it is and get Alex the directions. We hit the stairs to the garage (working smarter not harder), and make our way to ground level and head out. We step off and the Cadre stops us, and the clock. Why? Group pictures at the Hall of Fame of course! Ok, NOW we head out. Everyone is tired, everyone is sore, but spirits are high and the weights are moving around in good time, everyone getting a break when needed and jokes come a little more frequently now. We make the time hack with no problem. Reward: Go get some fatty treats, take a piss, and sit down. We have 15 minutes. I'm starting to get excited...

Get back to Freedom Park" - Time Hack 45 Minutes

Motivation for Current and Aspiring Endurance Challenge Athletes

Freedom Park...The start, end, start again and now the final end of two incredible challenges. We are heading there now! We gear up, grab the team weights and hit the greenway. It leads straight to the park so all we had to do was follow the walkway and not fall into the water! We had no problem making this time hack and we marched on towards the original start point from the edge of the park. The sun was just starting to rise, brand new dawn and hopefully the end of a very hard challenge.

WRONG!

Surprise! We are informed that we are nowhere NEAR close to being done. We grab the logs that Class 413 had used at their smoke session and marched off into a different part of the park...right towards where the F3 Class was gathered. The classes were grouped together in a big formation and instructed to break out into five even rows. We are then sent off to a different kind of Cadre Session. We are informed that those five even rows are now groups that are going to rotate between waiting cadre stationed throughout the park.

Station One: Cadre Patrick - Bounding Buddy team rushes, up a flipping snow covered hill! Then get on your stomach, turn around, put your feet on your butt and crawl back down the hill using just your arms.
Again...Again...Again. Push-ups, flutter kicks. Typical Patrick, it SUCKED!

Station Two: Cadre Rich - Pick your Poison. We got in a big circle, cadre in the center, and he points to someone, who picked an exercise and how many to do. He jacks up the number and everyone performs the exercise. Never once did Cadre Rich raise his voice. Very intimidating dude.

Station Three: Cadre "" - Suicide Drills using the parking lines in the parking lot (meaning a shit load of times back and forth). This was when my left ankle decided not to work anymore. I hobbled through the whole thing, falling WAY behind everyone else. I was maybe three fourths of the way done and everyone else was finished and staring at me. I basically just looked at the ground, gritted my teeth and finished the exercise. People patting me on the back giving me words of encouragement. Dan Husser from class 192 who finished long before me, jumped back in and finished up with me to help me out. Dude is awesome. A few more stupid F3 drills and we are on to the next area.

Station Four: Cadre Dan - Log PT. Ok. This sucked balls. All of the people took turns rotating through logs and rucks that had been set up and waiting for us. Some logs were big enough to fit six people under them, others had three, some just a single person. If you were not on a log, you were using a ruck. Non-stop fun here. The drill was over head, alternating log press, log squats, log abs, elevated pushups on the logs, flutter kicks with feet above the logs. Rotate! With Dan saying "Hurry up hurry up hurry up" constantly. Reps followed a pyramid pattern that ended up becoming more or less random according to how Dan was feeling at the time. Added bonus...the area we did this in was probably some kind of unofficial dog shitting area. Good times.

Station Five: Cadre Bert - Elephant walks and Find your rucksack game. You all know elephant walks, it was the same drill as the parking garage only with different people; we still managed to get it knocked out relatively quickly. The Find your ruck Game was interesting. We got ourselves into a line, set our rucks down in front of us, and then moved three or four people to the right. We were instructed to grab whatever ruck was in front of you and then get into a tight circle facing outwards. Bert yelled "Go!", and we ran outwards in a kind of starburst until he said stop, then we dropped the ruck and came back to the circle. He then gave us thirty seconds to find OUR original ruck (not the one we plopped in the field) and get back to the circle. This took a few tries and some head scratching on teamwork until we figured out how to do it without screwing each other over. Easy? Not really. It took us five tries to get it right. We stand around and bullshit for a bit and then head back to the main group...looks like we are now done.

We get back into a group with everyone (all ninety something of us); we take a group picture thinking we are going to head back to our start point for the big finish. Well, something like that happened, we grab our coupons and start marching back...but Dan and Bert veer off back towards the greenway. Sure enough, just like Cadre Dan said, "Everyone gets wet in a Challenge". So we enter the greenway under a bridge that consists of a sidewalk next to a deep stream strewn with broken concrete slabs and are then told that if we can do one good squat in unison (With all eighty F3 guys and Cadre Patrick watching) we would be done. Well into the water we went; three imperfect squats later we are done; cold, very wet and very happy. We head back up the ramp to the park and give high fives to the F3 group as we pass (they are lined up to be ordered into the water by Cadre Patrick. They have it rough now. Their start point is three miles down the road while ours is just over the hill.

We get to the finish finally! Patches are handed out; beers are enjoyed and hugs are going around. We never missed a time hack and they were very impressed with this. Cadre Dan makes a comment about me saying he doesn't want to hear about me doing B2B anymore, and I better be doing a Heavy and/or Selection soon. Both he and Bert are calling me a bad ass and tough as nails. It feels good to hear it from those guys. I took that second patch and just held it in my hand. No shit, I was near tears. I had just finished a B2B challenge and came out smiling and still walking. All the rucking (45 plus miles it turns out) over the last 24 hours was finally over with and I had survived.

One more round of pictures with the Cadre and team and a few more handshakes and I am heading home for a much needed shower and sleep.

Now to get ready to do this again in Boston HAHA!

Thanks for reading this, I hope you enjoyed it. I'm glad I wrote it down. In my advancing years, I am sure to forget a lot of this information in no time.

Todd 'Patches' Kruse.

Todd's story gives us some insight into what it takes to undertake a challenge that spans over twenty four hours with just enough rest and nourishment to make you always aware of how much pain you are in. As we have seen before preparation is key and motivation is a must for keeping spirits high during the most grueling parts of the challenge. Especially for Goruck events it can be all about the people to your left and right as there will likely be times when you cannot simply muscle through it and will need their help.

An event like a B2B Challenge is where your endurance training and event nutrition really shine. In an event this long and continuously stressful you will reach muscle fatigue and it will all be about your preparation and nutritional intake during the event to keep the intense muscle cramping and 'bonking' at bay. You can also gather from his story that events like this are what you make of them regarding your interactions with people and the

outcomes of events as the cadre assess whether or not you

are 'putting out' or holding back.

The First Goruck Heavy

Replying to desperate cries for more punishment Goruck cadre beta tested a 24+ hour event at Ft. Bragg with 73 enthusiastic participants. Designed to twice the intensity of the Goruck Challenge and then some the expectations were high. Every participant carries between 30 and 45lbs of personal gear and weight in their rucksack and shares another couple of hundred pounds of bonus objects between the class as a whole (logs, refrigerators, couches, PVC pipes filled with concrete etc.). These classes routinely push for more than 40 miles covered during the time period with many exceeding 50 or more.

Goruck is known for events that push participant's mental and physical boundaries with unconventional structure and team based challenges. In other events it is possible to go into your own personal happy place and 'push through it' so to speak; but can you perform as part of a team while doing this? Most people have to remain conscious and attentive in order to interact productively with others; this adds a whole new dimension to physical challenge. David Kim learned this lesson first hand when he was assigned as team leader of a whole squad of participants at the very first Goruck Heavy at Ft. Bragg North Carolina:

David Kim:

The unofficial theme of the inaugural Heavy was leadership. How it cascades down from the top but it must also well from the bottom up too. Bottom line, everyone has to step up. GRTs know this. But put this to the test over 24 hours of grueling long movements filled with casualties, coupon retrievals, punishment smoke-fests, and the over-engineering of cadre-sanctioned bathroom breaks, even Selectees need remedial training that sometimes needs to be learned through pain and suffering. Given that our class was laden with GRT all-stars, teamwork and morale were high in the beginning. But as night turned into day we came to a baseball field where decimation awaited us.

We all know that smoke fests are part of the deal, but I think the tempo and duration of what Cadre Patrick put us through was a shock for some. You could literally see it on people's faces. "Too cold, too wet, too muddy, too tired, too much, too long, I'm done." People were dropping like flies.

But time, distance, and crushing weight soon started to take its toll as everything became noticeably more of a struggle as we trudged on. Yes, physically it was draining but no matter how physically excruciating it was, there was never a moment in my mind where I thought of quitting. Of course it helps when you have teammates looking out for you. Thank you guys! But let's not kid ourselves, the waxing and waning of selflessness and selfishness that is the inherent crucible in a GRC can make or break a class and this maxim was certainly amplified a thousand fold in our Heavy.

Case in point, I was losing focus near the end because I was focusing more on my own personal survival than looking out for my squad and the class. At that point, I was in a Selection frame of mind, i.e. individual survival, don't be last, physically perform kind of mode and not really thinking team. Big mistake.

During the last night movement, Cadre asked me if everyone on my squad was accounted for. I started to count off and....two men are missing. $%#$@!!! A search party went out to look for my missing squad members and I was promptly fired as Squad Leader. What I didn't know was that Cadre instructed my two squad members who took a bathroom break during our last long movement to intentionally hide out to test the situational awareness of the leadership and I failed miserably because I became a zombie. Because of me the class indexed with a smoke fest rather than take cool guy pictures at an SF monument that was ours to be had.

Don't get me wrong, our Heavy was by no means a bummer. "We rise and fall together as a team!" and "you weren't the only set of eyes who didn't notice missing teammates" my class swiftly reminded me. There were so many awesome thrilling moments our class had such as visiting many of monuments of our greatest SOF heroes, getting a private tour of the JFKSWCS, log PT in the Pit, bearing witness to Cadre Dan's reenlistment, and earning the ODA 3336's coin.

I got to ruck with my GRT friends old and new as well as a rare opportunity to ruck with my Selection bros all at once. All my wishes were fulfilled and next to earning my Selection patch, it is my greatest Goruck memory yet. The reason why, perhaps best expressed by Cadre Garrett's AAR of our class because his frank and poignant feedback was the ultimate reward:

"We train to standard, not time. As you all know, the event went on for 24.5 hours. That last half hour was because the team fucked up, SPECIFICALLY the leadership. We had a couple of cool stops to see before the end, like the USASOC memorial and 3rd Group memorial. Both humbling tear jerking emotional but awesome sights to see that immortalize our greatest heroes. But because you guys fucked up, we had to use the remainder of the time for "education" purposes.

In Goruck you get rewarded no matter what, whether it is seeing cool stuff, learning through humble pie, or learning through pain and misery. It is always up to the class. Other than that last two hours, I thought you guys did outstanding. But it's when you are most tired, most hungry, and most complacent when shit happens and people die. Don't let your buddies die. There is no greater regret in this world or the next as far as I'm concerned. Great to see you all again! Cheers!"

I (the author) also had the pleasure of being at Bragg Heavy as it has come to be known. The stress and strain put on the participants multiplied the fatigue and weariness one would normally feel staying up for 24 straight hours. Being part of a team and more importantly a team leader during this time was such a challenge precisely because you had to focus on others besides yourself and put their needs before your own. Learning how to lead when the chips are down and you are out of your comfort zone is invaluable and Kim and I would recommend it to anyone even remotely interested. This kind of experience goes so far beyond the standard race format that anyone looking to break out of 'running K's' should

Motivation for Current and Aspiring Endurance Challenge Athletes
Vol. 1 332

look into it.

Bragg Heavy 2.0 AAR

By: James Vreeland

Preface: While this event is not as secretive as Selection, there are elements to the evolutions/methods of the Cadre that are best experienced for one's self. For that reason, several aspects of this AAR will be intentionally vague/redacted. As a civilian, being on base and standing on the fields and grounds whose names I've known for years was a unique and emotional honor. I'll just get the confession out of the way now, I got a little weepy on a number of occasions. Sue me.

-18h

I arrived in town Thursday night and decide to forego the few ruckoffs around town. I figured I would have plenty of time to catch up with friends (new and old) on the trail

-12h

Left hotel and met up with a few other Michigan GRTs that I planned on suffering with. We didn't know how squads would be determined, but we figured if we stayed in proximity to each other early on, the chances of being grouped together for the duration would go up. We spent some time game-planning, shuffling gear around to get ruck weight dialed in, set up a few contingencies for how we would ideally handle some challenges we expected to be faced with (loss of talking privileges, how to quickly group people by like weights/heights, etc), and filled our guts with high calorie rocket fuel at Cracker Barrel.

-8h

First things first, slip on to post and talk your way in to the Green Beret Club to have a few beers with Cadre ██████, where you are told that you are an idiot for even attempting this challenge.

A number of people had made plans to tour the Airborne & Special Operations Museum, so we met out front, took a group photo out front and began our tour. The mood was friendly, but it was very obvious that people were already churning their guts and trying to be mentally prepared for the next day and a half. Almost immediately my mental gameplan was thrown out the window when I turned a corner and came face to face with the wreckage of Super 61 - http://i.imgur.com/KJGPJuf.png - http://en.wikipedia.org/wiki/Battle_of_Mogadishu_(1993).

It became very clear that I would be encountering many things over the next few days that I was simply not expecting to see in my lifetime. Cue weepy moment #1. After the tour a few of us set off for food and stumbled into Cadre ██████████. We convinced him to join us for a last meal and tried valiantly to pump him for intel. No such luck, just evil smiles.

-4h

Back to the hotel to rack out. I'm terrible at napping unless I'm dead tired, so this was just time where I laid still and spaced out for a bit, sent my "I'm going dark, see you on the other side" texts, and generally tried to relax.

-2h

Woke up the group, loaded out cars, moved towards the start point. Credentials were checked at the gate, we were moving across base, this was now a very real thing. We arrived at the start point and waiting in vehicles until checked in by Cadre. Unloaded gear, made the rounds saying "hi" to folks I've met over time, snuck out to the fence line to try to piss out the nerves. It didn't work.

0h (all future times are estimates)

"Hurry up, we're already behind schedule. Get over there in ranks. Hurry up, don't be last. Why are you moving so damn slowly?" Oh hi Cadre Dan.

Rules and expectations for the event were set out. Holy crap there were a lot of Cadre milling around. PT tests for pushups and situps were run, following age/gender rules of the APFT. I've always done "crossfit" push ups where the chest (only chest, no thighs) lightly taps the ground for a split second to mark the bottom of the rep, I've never heard otherwise as a requirement. I was *fortunate* enough to have Jason judging my reps and he was having none of this style and he immediate starting laying in to me about my form. Not sure if he really cared about my technique or Cadre were just making examples of people early on to sow seeds of fear. Either way, it worked and threw me for a second. Good job. While waiting for your turn to PT, groups faced away and stood quietly. My column was on the leading edge into the wind, so we all started getting chilly right off the bat.

After PT was ruck inspection and weigh in. Don't be light. More targets were painted on people for violations. Use the sand pit to get up to weight, quickly. Dan briefed us on the next event, the 12 mile road ruck march. Headlamps on, mouths shut. Move with a purpose over the course. Don't be last. Dan would be setting *a* pace, but gave no indication of what speed that would be. Flags up front, you must be back here in under 3:30, go.

By the way, take all the food out of your pack and dump it into the Kit Bags up at the front of the ranks. No calories for the foreseeable future. This was definitely an individual event, but I'm decent at gauging pace, so I worked with my desired teammates to set a quick enough hustle to keep us well ahead of the hack/scrutiny, but just slow enough to keep us all together. We finished in 2:20, but I think the course was a hair shorter than 12 due to road construction. None the less, we were cruising.

+5h

As we came in from the ruck we were broken into squads and told to get in formation, fix our issues, shut up, and wait for further instructions. Our initial prep work paid off as all of the folks I came to this event with made it into Squad 4. We took this time to refit on water, fix feet, get some weight off of our feet. Once all rosters were off the course squads were assigned team weights (we got: the food bags ~100# x2, a sandbag ~80#, two water jugs ~50# x2), and broken off in different directions. An LMTV pulled up and Squad 1 loaded up and were taken off. We were now basically waiting our turn to get packed up and moved on to base. Our lead cadre was Dakotah with Cadre Joe as his second, and he felt this temporary delay was the ideal time to start a Welcome Party.

What felt like 2 hours later it was finally our turn to load up in the truck and move on. Rucks/weights in the trailer, bodies in the back of the truck. Shut up, lamps off, don't you dare peek out the sides of the truck. Charlie Mike.

The truck came to a stop and we unloaded ...somewhere. There were a couple people on my team from the 82nd and they mentioned that we were ~10 miles from our staging area. We then began a series of long movements with time hacks. The team weights were pretty nasty, and struggled to keep pace. I think we blew most of the hacks. We moved for hours, and honestly I couldn't tell you exactly when, but we picked up some bonus coupons along the way (ammo cans full of sand ~40# x2, weapons crates full of sand ~60# x2, a handleless crate full of god knows what ~180#).

For those keeping score at home, our squad of 23 now had a flag and 10 coupons. Some time before we took on the big crate we got hit with heavy casualties for missing a hack and had every set of hands on either bodies or coupons for about a mile. We moved under oppressive load for a long time, which is honestly my favorite way to suffer through these things. I'd rather be an ox than soaking in a freezing river at night. Not sure when, but it must have been near sunrise as we saw the occasional human moving around, we were tasked with 15 ascents of a series of stairs with all of our gear.

This task frayed the nerves of more than one sleepyhead but we all made it through and carried on, after about 90 minutes. Unfortunately, shortly after the steps our group suffered a med drop. An ammo can slipped during a transition and cracked someone in the head, they were actively attempting to continue, but after exhibiting signs of a concussion cadre made the call and pulled them from the event. You can patch up busted feet, hydrate away minor heat exhaustion, but there sadly nothing that can be done for blunt force head trauma on the move.

Every once in a while Cadre would stop us and give us the "do you know where you are?" test, which in almost every instance we did not. Most of the time we were then informed of the hallowed ground we were standing on, and the significance of the area (graduation grounds where every member of ▮▮▮▮▮▮▮ has stood, SWC school, memorial to ▮▮▮▮). Cue weepy moments #2+.

At some point after sunrise we had moved far/not far enough, done well/poor enough to dump sand from some of the coupons, load the empties in to a truck and begin moving with a purpose towards our next objective, Pike Field. We were down to 3 coupons and the jerry cans of water.

+14h

We got there, last, and saw the other three squads taking some downtime for beating their hack. This was not to be our fate. To make up for missing our hacks we did rounds of PT broken up by team sprints around a downfield target, with more time hacks. Miss your time, the round did not count. You win some, you lose some, eventually the exercise ends. Our group got a few minutes to refit **AND EAT**. We did some quick damage to that feed bag before Dan came front and center to introduce a surprise guest. The translator attached to Cadre Doug's unit was on hand to tell the story of his experiences and of how he moved his family to the States. It was a story of the wars often overlooked as almost all focus on the operations abroad relates to US forces, and leaves out the bravery of the local elements that make the jobs of our soldiers possible.

+16h

Rucks on, starting moving out as a team. The easy part is over. Who wants to hop in the truck and have some of these delicious donuts and warm coffee? HURRY UP.

People who had done the event at Bragg last year immediately stopped smiling because they "knew" where we heading. I try to make it a point to not make guesses at what is coming next. Staying in the moment helps keep my mind in the right place. With that said, if you have spent hours in small groups, recently shed weight, combined forces, and are marching towards the Log PT area - chances are good it is time to put logs over head.

There isn't much to say about the next three or four hours, except that it looked like http://i.imgur.com/gYVznfv.jpg and http://i.imgur.com/VmxRaU3.jpg. Your group is screwing up the motions during log PT, or simply too slow? They must be overheating, get in the pond.

Oh, and three people were pulled out of the water area with stage two hypothermia. Cadre on the sidelines had a pretty good idea of who in the group had experience in dealing with getting people back in the game, as issues became evident folks (myself included) were voluntold to drag those in danger out of the water and over for med checks and to get them into a safe state. Nothing like stripping down in the bed of a truck with a stranger who is fighting you because they are panicking and in fear of being med-dropped to get the blood flowing. I brought my "patient" back to coherence and was directed over to log pit to warm up myself.

After enough soak time Dan called it quits on our bath time and directed everyone over to the pit and instructed us to wring out gear and start to warm up. We got a second chance at calories, and ate greedily.

protip: impromptu dance parties are a great way to get blood circulation going again. no one is going to judge your actions after nearly a day on the move. I totally won't heckle teammates for years to come regarding their terrible moves.

+20h

We were given time to get dry/warm enough to continue then Dan rolled up in a HMMWV (one of the benefits of being on Bragg is the toys), combined squads to make two large groups then played "follow the armored vehicle through the woods". As it turns out, military vehicles can roll through some pretty ugly terrain, so we did as well.

One of the canons of the new Heavy SOP is that this is to be the ultimate team event. Our next evolution put this to the test as elements of Robin Sage and "the apparatus" were combined. Teams had to gain the permission and support of "indigenous forces" (cadre) to move through their lands and utilize supplies from their camp to design and build carts to drag newer, heavier coupons down the trail. If you've seen the movie "2 weeks in hell", these devices should look familiar - http://i.imgur.com/hoRCaPQ.jpg.

The local leader require us to perform a celebratory dance to show respect for their culture before we could continue. Now, I'm not an expert in Civil Affairs or local culture, but the dance sure seemed to bear many similarities to "a boatload of burpees".

We got our gear and began designing solutions. It is important to note that there is no really *good* solution possible given the supplies at your disposal. The exercise is designed to force teams to work well under stressful situations, the best you can hope for is an acceptably bad solution that survives brute force. Ours did and my squad pulled ahead and stayed there. "It pays to be a winner", right? Not this time. Since we were so far ahead of the group behind us, cadre decided that we had to turn around and regroup with the other squad.

Tempers flared, but we kept the rage in check and continued the exercise. By this point the sun was setting, so we knew two things with certainty a) we had been moving for nearly 24 hours and b) no one wanted to drag these horrible carts over rough terrain in the dark. Fires were lit under asses and we made go time in reforming with the other group.

Somehow it was decided that we were too clean/dry/warm (none of these things were really true, but that doesn't matter), so the squads were ordered to form opposing ranks in knee deep mud and run "indirect fire" drills - aka: face the woods and throw handfuls of mud at the poor sucker behind you, mortar-style. Once we were gross and cold again we were allowed to continue towards a new target location, the log pit. We moaned and started to hustle, my squad broke away in the lead again. We reached the pond and were cleared to dump the weight out of our coupons and break down the apparatus. This trudge just turned into a race, and we were not about to lose. Ever seen 40 zombies jog in formation with a couple dozen pieces of gear shouldered? It's a sight to behold.

+26h

Our squad reached a wooded park and stacked up the gear behind the LMTV and got back into formation. Dakotah and Joe split us in to two teams and mine took off on a fast march down the road. We made a big loop and cycled back to where we parted ways with the others, who were now gone. Orders were given to use the water station to rinse off rucks and bodies, then get back into formation. Rucks were loaded in to the trailer, bodies in the truck and we were off down the road.

+28h

The truck slammed to a stop, we were bullhorned out of the back, and ordered to lay out all gear in formation then start lining up drop bags we turned in at the beginning of the event; also in formation. Cadre made it **very** clear that the event was not over and we could be dropped at any time, so zero screwing around as we washed down gear, stowed it, and awaited the second squad - who had to ruck halfway back to the start point as a penalty for losing to us in the race. They finally arrived, serviced their gear and Dan lined us up in formation.

+30h

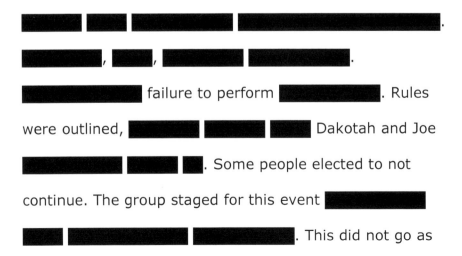

███████ ███ ████████ ██████████████████████████.
█████████, ███, ███████████ ██████████.
███████████ failure to perform ██████████. Rules were outlined, ██████ █████ ███ Dakotah and Joe ████████ ██████ █. Some people elected to not continue. The group staged for this event ██████████ ████ █████████████ ████████████. This did not go as

expected, as expected. ████████ ██ ███████; █████████ ██████ ██. Direction was given to stop, and we were done. We were endexed. GRH 027 was in the books.

Roughly 120 started the event, nearly 90 completed.

Motivation for Current and Aspiring Endurance Challenge Athletes

Baptism By Fire

Lauren Cisneros

HEAVY 030 NYC 4/4/14:

17,000+ calories burned

26.5 hours

47+ miles

41lb ruck

78 registered, 59 started, 42 finished

I can't go without typing up what I went through this weekend. Not all of you will understand why I went through this. I trained my butt off, spent a good amount of money on it and had no intentions of changing my mind. Some things are unexplainable. Here is my story.

"What the hell is GORUCK?"

I learned about GORUCK about a year ago during the NJ Super Spartan Hurricane Heat. It's where I met Steve-o, Jeremy and Henry -- some of the most inspiring people I know. It is also where I became a part of an amazing team called Team Braveheart in which we inspire others to be brave! Jen Rosant – the leader of Braveheart is such an inspiration. I have never been part of a team with such amazing individuals. At every event that I participate in I wear my black and red kilt to represent my team.

During the Hurricane Heat in NJ –a lot of participants had these "backpacks" as I called them, on and I was confused as to why they all had the same type of pack. They continued to tell me about this team building event called GORUCK and the requirement of having to have 35 pounds of weight in your ruck, dry during a HEAVY which is a 24+ hour event. Throughout the Hurricane Heat (another type of team event) Steve-o, JB and Henry kept telling me about how I should sign up for a GORUCK event with them as it is the ultimate team building event. I loved every minute of that Hurricane Heat with those guys and knew I had to do something similar, if not more. I loved working as a team, putting others first and working together towards completing the mission at hand.

Steve-o and several others who I met through Spartan mentioned to me they were signed up for the HEAVY (24 hour + ultimate team building event) on April 4th. I contemplated signing up -- but wasn't sure. I would have never thought that I would ever sign myself up for a 24 hour event, never mind my first GORUCK event ever. It isn't cheap to do one of these events with the gear you need, food, etc. I am forever grateful to Derek for helping me get to the HEAVY. Not sure I could have done it otherwise. The GORUCK community has such an amazing group of people that help each other out no matter the circumstances. In January of this year I officially signed up and had exactly 2.5 months to train my butt off. This is when it got real.

On my 21st birthday (Feb 2nd) I didn't spend it by going out to the bar for a few drinks; I instead joined a bunch of fellow Bravehearts who I never had met before on a 12 mile ruck on Sandy Hook, NJ. Jeanette, Dave, and Joey helped me train hard and got me ready for the toughest event of my life. I'll never forget the 4 hour philosophical conversation I had with Jeanette while Dave and Joey went ahead at a quicker pace. To keep things light we had a hilarious photo session at the end of Sandy Hook where the nude beach sign is.

That's when I knew I had made the right 21st birthday decision -- spend it with people that are as crazy as I am and are some of the most positive people I know. I trained hard for this event, but I could have trained harder. With being a full time college student and working all the time, it was extremely difficult to fit long rucks in. I started off with a 20# ruck and gradually increased my weight to 50# about a month before the event.

I did a lot of cross training, running, started crossfit, etc -- was glad that I was REALLY comfortable with pushups, burpees and sit ups before this event. Would have been extremely hard (even more so than it was) to complete the event with all of the PT we were put through. Everyone seems to train differently. Do what works for you. So many people worry about the PT test but really, it should be the least of your concerns. You won't be dropped for failing the PT.

I think one of my biggest concerns before this event was, "should I bring this, should I buy that? What shoes should I wear?!" A typical newbie GR moment. Some people I reached out to said that during their heavy, the cadres took away their food -- others said that in their class the cadres let them keep theirs. My heavy was 26.5 hours -- I believe I ate 2 builders bars, 2 clif bars, some dark chocolate espresso beans, clif blocks, my water with fUS and nothing else.

We only got one break for 15 minutes at a gas station in the middle of Brooklyn somewhere around 6-7am. I was shocked that I was able to push myself for as long as I did with what seems like such little food – but when your body is screaming and you're focused on the mission, eating is one of the last things that comes to mind.

Footwear was also another big concern for me in which I thought I had it down pat. This HEAVY made me realize that with all the training I did, I never trained my feet as much as I should have. Two days post HEAVY and my feet are really bad. Three toenails are gone, blisters everywhere. I wore Asics that were one size bigger than I usually wear to allow for swelling. I thought my feet would be perfect, but they are far from that a few days post. Learn from me and make sure you include proper foot care in your training!

I thought about quitting.. several times.. but I didn't quit. I trained hard for this -- I wanted this, I was part of a team that needed me. It was about always putting the mission first. We became one unit, one team. One person suffered, we all suffered. No matter how much pain I was in, I knew someone else was in just as much, if not more pain than I was. 1/3 through the event I pulled my inner thigh and zombie walked the entire event in pain. We went 47.5 miles from Coney Island to Central Park carrying our 40# ruck, and our team weight of a 50# steel apple, 50# sandbag, 80# sandbag and 100# sandbag.

I quickly realized that mental strength mattered more than physical strength as it took all of my mental capacity to focus on the mission at hand. Every time my team didn't cross at the pedestrian crossing within the seconds given before the "walking man" symbol disappears, Cadre Geoff made sure we suffered a great amount of PT for it. Our team quickly learned to cross streets safely, as a unit, and at a fast pace.

The cadre were amazing -- Cadre Jason, Geoff, and Big Daddy -- some of the finest cadre GR has to offer. We started with 59 and ended with 42 brave souls. Our class was split during the trek to Central Park from about 4am to around noon. Cadre Geoff was with my team the entire time until we "lost" him at a quick bathroom break at a local firehouse. He continuously asked us what the flag represents. I never even thought about what the red, white and blue stood for. After some more PT -- I will never forget that the 50 stars represent the states, the 13 stripes represent the colonies, the red -- valour, the white -- purity, and the blue -- vigilance, perseverance and justice. GR is all about making better Americans.

We went through hell and back to earn our patches.

Several PT sessions which included flutter kicks, wall sits with our 40# rucks over our heads, beach sprint, beach low crawls, 8 count bodybuilders, push-ups, squats, lunges... the list continues. Our 12 mile ruck on the beach turned into a 20 mile rainy, wet, ruck that made most of us realize that this was not a walk in the park by any means. My teammates didn't let me quit -- they helped me push through the pain even though I thought there was nothing left in me.

I was thankful I brought pink sunglasses with me -- I may have looked cool, but behind those sunglasses was a stream of tears down my face. Cadre John aka (Big Daddy) calmed me down and reminded me to put the mission first once we reached Central Park. I was breaking down at that point, but once he finished telling us the importance of teamwork and always putting the mission first, I was able to shut my mind off and all the pain went away.

I was honored to become TL (team leader) and lead the team to the next mission, and the finish point. We had to find "downed pilots" in the park which were actually 2 logs -- one was probably 100# or so approximately which the ladies took and the other was a legitimate tree. It took about 30 of our men to carry that log up a hill to our finish point. It was so inspiring and amazing to see everyone give it all they had to finish that mission. We reached the top of that hill, and saw a monument with the American flag dancing in the wind.

We were instructed to sing the Star Spangled Banner and the National Anthem (I had to conduct.. haha). After that, all 3 Cadre came together to announce that we had completed the NYC HEAVY. At that moment, a wave of relief came over us. We did it. We rucked 26.5 hours, 47.5 miles. 59 of us started 42 of us finished. My first GORUCK was in the books. NYC HEAVY #030 completed. I was in shock. I still am.

I never thought I would complete such an emotional, physical, and all around taxing journey. Who would of thought the fat kid in middle school would become an endurance athlete? GORUCK is a new chapter in my life and I am happy to be a part of the GRT community. Never think any challenge is too great to accomplish...you might surprise yourself!

So.. what are you waiting for? Sign up for some good livin'! Oh, and Always. Look. Cool.

Lauren Cisneros -- AKA "The woman in the schoolgirl outfit".

Back to Back to Back to Back Endurance Challenges

By: Chris Holt

GORUCK HCLS Class 001:

I'm pretty sure I'm not supposed to be here. I mean, I actually signed up for the Challenge in Boulder this day, as an excuse to get on a plane and visit friends out West. Then one thing led to another, plans got kyboshed, and Jason told us all we needed to be in Jacksonville. So here I am, packed in the Mystery Machine with the youthful and well bearded Adam, and the steely eyed and surprisingly tall Grant, hurtling at impressive speeds (this is a lie) directly towards HCLS in Jacksonville Florida (this is the truth). We stop for a break for some primo pre-event nutrition at Sonic. 30 minutes later my stomach feels queasy, yet I can't discern if it is from the grease mortar that just shot down my throat, or if it is because what I am about to do is sinking in.

HCLS stands for Heavy, Challenge, Light, Scavenger. Wearing a pack weighted with bricks and other gear, we will participate in a team based endurance challenge that is supposed to last 24 hours (Heavy), 12 hours (Challenge), and 6 hours (Light). Given GORUCKs penchant to under promise and over deliver, I am fairly confident that at least one of these events will run over (I am right). The schedule allows for a few hours of rest between the Heavy and the Challenge, and another few hours between the Challenge and the Light. Following the Light is an actual full night of sleep, leading into a 2 hour un-weighted Scavenger hunt.

Grant, Adam and I arrive Wednesday night late and crash in a hotel room. Grant, who is a big fan of free breakfast spreads, wakes us all up to trudge downstairs for the best that Hampton Inn has to offer. We gorge ourselves, return to the room, and immediately pass out until right before our late checkout.

A few hours and some last minute shopping later we are at the start point for the Heavy. The Cadre show up a few minutes after we do, and they are ready for business.

We form up, weigh rucks, and start with the PT test. 49 pushups and 59 situps in 2 minutes each? No problem. I have been training for the GORUCK Selection standard of 55 and 65, so I breeze through these. Not so for Fat Joel. He can't make the 49, so we all rest while he gives another attempt. It pays to be a winner. (Note: Joel does not appear to actually be fat. But he does suck at pushups. We would ridicule him more for this, but he did most of the HCLS in flip flops which in my opinion makes him a badass. And a nutjob).

We immediately start the 12 mile ruck, performed this time as a group. Cadre Dakotah sets an approximately 15 min/mile pace, which keeps us hustling. Within the first two miles I start noticing hot spots on the balls of my feet. Ruh Roh. This is a problem. I have tested this shoe/sock combination before for long rucks so I am not sure what this is about… maybe the humidity… maybe this specific pace/stride is just unnatural for me and is causing issues. Hard to say. Just keep moving.

The rest of the Heavy is pretty standard for a GORUCK event, although I will say that this one felt extra Heavy (I have only done one other, so not a ton to compare it to). Cadre loaded us up with sand filled kegs, giant sand filled balls, and more sandbags than I care to remember. We covered a big chunk of Jacksonville on foot, and ended with a run. This turned into another issue for me, as my hot spots had turned into legit blisters and my knees are starting to hurt (this happens every time I run with a ruck). 30 of the 35 that started get patched about 26 hours later, and have just over 2 hours to eat, change, and prep for the Challenge. No sleep will be had this night. Adam, Grant and I head straight for fuel depot #2: Five Guys. I can barely walk as I place my order and return to my seat. Adam lets loose the thought that he was really just concerned with completing the Heavy. He doesn't really need to do the rest of this. EXACTLY what I wanted to hear. I just need to cosign his BS and the two of us can frolic around Jacksonville while Grant and the rest of these weirdos stay up all night (again).

I think about a great blog post I read last week about getting your mind right with training. One of the tips the author gave was basically to just suit up and show up for training with the idea he could always quit later. 90% of the time when he did this he would end up staying and completing the workout and would be glad that he did. I was legitimately doubting my ability to actually finish the next event given my knee pain, but I decided to just change, ruck up, and see what happens. I vaguely remember Grant telling Adam to just shut up and get ready, and before I know it we are all at the start of the Challenge along with 10 other Heavy finishers.

My prediction was that the Challenge would be the toughest of the 3 events to get through. I was right. We headed straight to the beach, and had our Welcome Party (intense exercise smoke session) in the surf. It was dark. Waves were crashing over us and strewing us across the sand. Cadre were shining flashlights in our faces and yelling. There were 4 or 5 Cadre present, but it felt like we each had our own. Annmarie described the Welcome Party as "almost scary," which I feel was a pretty apt descriptor.

I am just starting to think I won't be able to finish this when I see one of the 13 get up and walk away, shouting something like "screw this crap it's too effin cold." Now we are down to 12. Something clicks, and I know I am not following him out of the surf. We start low crawling as a group, face in the mud, looking for some object in the surf that may or may not even be there, and I realize that I am actually enjoying this. I am having fun.

The Challenge goes all night. It feels every bit as heavy as the Heavy. We carry Cadre Aaron down the beach on a couch, which stays with us all night, along with pretty much everything that we carried during the Heavy. It's heavy. It sucks. I hurt. But I know at this point that I am not quitting. No matter what.

We all start getting really tired around hour 6 of the Challenge. Every time we stop for any reason I see Adam and Grant actually sleeping on their feet. At one point Cadre Joel takes us through some stupid # of calf raises (like 250), and I watch Adam complete about 5 calf raises while actually asleep. I can verify this as he was snoring slightly.

The Challenge runs over at about 14 hours, and we are told we have an hour and 15 minutes to get ready for the Light. GR ends up pushing the start time back 1 hour, but there still is not time to sleep. We DO have time for a quick rinse off in the outdoor shower at GR HQ, which was a real game changer. There was also an angel that showed up at the Light start point with cheeseburgers for those of us that didn't have time to stop for food.

As soon as we form up for the Light, I know this event will be a totally different story. Cadre Dakotah gets up in front of all of us with a huge shit eating grin, and all kinds of crap is given to the now 3 Selection finishers who are doing the Light with us. As promised, the Light is not Easy, but it is a heck of a lot of fun. We carry large rubber Zodiac boats to a beach and proceed to play Pirates of the Carribean with them, ramming each other's boats and throwing eggs in lieu of firing canons. This was quite possible the best time I have had at a GORUCK event. Songs were sung, topless runners were applauded, and smiles were in abundance.

The Light ended with a party at GR HQ, and then we hit up our hotel for the night. Sunday we stumbled to the pier for a 2 hr speed Scavenger, and were dismayed to find we had to earn a certain # of points in order to get our HCLS patch. No hiding out for these 2 hours. Instead, we enlisted the help of 1 Lifeguard, 2 little girls, 4 teenagers, and 2 Vietnam Vets in obtaining enough pictures of badassery and shenanigans to eventually place 2nd in this event. Of the 35 that started the Heavy, 12 finished: The Sandy Dozen. I will always and forever be grateful to each of these fine people, and for the opportunity to suffer through these 4 events with them.

Learnings from the event:

Mom's minivan really IS bitchin'. You likely will not have time to sleep between events at an HCLS, so don't bother with a hotel room for the nights of the Heavy and Challenge.

It's all about showing up. Of the 13 that showed up for the start of the Challenge, 12 finished the entire HCLS. So just suit up and show up.

Be prepared to walk through injury. I dealt with a bad knee starting at the end of the Heavy, and it bothered me for the rest of the event.

Getting off caffeine completely for a week before the events was pretty key. I did not need much in the way of caffeine supplements and seemed to be more awake than most during the Challenge.

Perfect nutrition for HCLS starts and ends with cheeseburgers. I had one before each event.

Flip flops MAY be the right boots for Selection.

Final Thoughts

I hope that you were able to bring benefit to yourself and your future endeavors with the collected information here. Again, I am not trying to stake a claim to new paradigms or push back the boundaries of exercise science/competition tactics. The entire premise of this work was simply to collect the opinions and experiences of accomplished athletes and give you (the reader) the ability to access it before undertaking the event in question. I hope this book helps you to reduce the number of times you have to learn 'the hard way', become experienced faster, and turn around and help someone else reach their goals.

Right, wrong, or indifferent, the opinions given by the athletes quoted in this book were developed through individual experience. Claiming that these opinions are universally beneficial to anyone and everyone would be silly. I encourage you to mull over what they had to say, rationalize their experiences and advice. Do your own research and testing and in the end come up with your own course of action, even if it is totally different. Also with regards to businesses mentioned in this work:

My summaries and evaluations (and those of those interviewed for this book) of them and their events are opinions only and do not reflect any official stance, mission statement, or overall goal of their company or intent for events and those who participate in them.

I am not sponsored by any of these companies and have received no financial compensation for mentioning them (or discussing them) in this work and neither have those interviewed here. All persons quoted in this work were either consulted directly and asked specifically for permission to publish their words or their opinions were openly sourced from freely accessible internet sources available to the general public at all times.

Source List and Recommended Reading

- Cordain, Loren. *The Paleo Diet for Athletes*. Rodale, 2012. EPUB file.

- Doneen, Nathan. *The Divide: A 2700 mile Search For Answers*. Author, 2014. EPUB file.

- Greenfield, Ben. *Rewriting the Fat Burning Textbook*. http://www.bengreenfieldfitness.com/2014/05/how-much-fat-can-you-burn/.

- Grylls, Bear. Mud, Sweat, and Tears. William Morrow, 2012. EPUB file.

- Jurek, Scott. *Eat and Run*. Mariner Books, 2013. Print.

- Mackenzie, *Brian. Power Speed ENDURANCE: A Skill-Based Approach to Endurance Training*. Victory Belt Publishing, 2013. EPUB file.

- Roach, Mary. *Gulp: Adventures on the Alimentary Canal*. W. W. Norton & Company, 2014. Audiobook.

- Rosenthal, Norman. *The Gift of Adversity: The Unexpected Benefits of Life's Difficulties, Setbacks, and*

Imperfections. Tarcher, 2013. EPUB file.

- Taubes, Gary. *Why We Get Fat and What To Do About It*. Anchor, 2011. Print.

- Teicholz, Nina. *The Big Fat Surprise*. S&S, 2014. Print.

- Tortorich, Vinnie. *Fitness Confidential*. Telemachus Press, 2013. Print.

- Viesturs, Ed. No Shortcuts to the Top. Broadway Books, 2006. EPUB file.

- Vonhof, John. *Fixing Your Feet: Prevention and Treatments for Athletes*. Wilderness press, 2011. EPUB file.

Made in the USA
Charleston, SC
11 July 2015